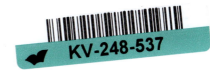

Medical Library
Downsizing
*Administrative, Professional,
and Personal Strategies
for Coping with Change*

Medical Library Downsizing

Administrative, Professional, and Personal Strategies for Coping with Change

Michael J. Schott, MA, MLS

The Haworth Information Press®
An Imprint of The Haworth Press
New York • London • Oxford

Published by

The Haworth Information Press®, an imprint of The Haworth Press, Inc., 10 Alice Street, Binghamton, NY 13904-1580.

PUBLISHER'S NOTE
The development, preparation, and publication of this work have been undertaken with great care. However, the publisher, employees, editors, and agents of The Haworth Press are not responsible for any errors contained herein or for consequences that may ensue from use of materials or information contained in this work. The opinions expressed by the author(s) are not necessarily those of The Haworth Press, Inc.

Cover design by Jennifer M. Gaska.

Library of Congress Cataloging-in-Publication Data

Schott, Michael J.
    Medical library downsizing: administrative, professional, and personal strategies for coping with change / Michael J. Schott.
        p. cm.
    Includes bibliographical references and index.
    ISBN 0-7890-0413-5 (alk. paper)—ISBN 0-7890-0420-8 (pbk. alk. paper)
1. Medical libraries—Administration. 2. Hospital libraries—Administration. 3. Medical libraries—Personnel management. 4. Hospital libraries—Personnel management. 5. Downsizing of organizations. 6. Organizational change. I. Title.
Z675.M4S36 2005
025.1'9661—dc22
                                                                                        2004012741

In loving memory of Diana Allan.
A great nurse, a great woman,
and the best person to have on your team
during a downsizing.

ABOUT THE AUTHOR

Michael Schott, MLS, MA, has worked at the West Virginia University Charleston Division since 2000. He is responsible for all operations of the health sciences library. Michael holds two master's degrees: an MA from Glassboro State University in New Jersey and an MLS from Southern Connecticut State University in Connecticut. Previously, he was the director of the Danbury Hospital (a 400-bed community teaching hospital) Library for 13 years and before that an Assistant Director of the health sciences library at New York Medical College in Valhalla, New York. Michael is an active writer. His works have appeared in *MLA News, CWIS* (Campus-Wide Information Systems), *Profiles* (the hospital marketing journal), and the *Journal of Hospital Librarianship*. Michael grew up in Margate, New Jersey, four blocks from the Atlantic Ocean. He presently lives in Hurricane, West Virginia.

CONTENTS

Preface   xi

Acknowledgments   xiii

Chapter 1. Introduction   1

Corporate View of Downsizing   4
Paradigm Shift Without a Clutch   5
Health Care Reality   6
Figures Don't Lie, Liars Figure   9
Definitions   10
The Nastiest Secret of All   13

Chapter 2. Arming Yourself (Before the Announcement)   17

Secret Arrow in the Quiver: The Résumé   18
Positive Power of Great Leadership   20
Sword in the Scabbard: The Mission Statement   21
Mace of Righteous: Your Management Style   24
Stout Shield of the Arm: Certifications and Regulations   25
Protective Helmet: The Numbers of Your Life   27
Greaves of Steel: Benchmarks, Flowcharts,
    Organization Charts, and Evaluation Surveys   29
More Arrows to Fill the Quiver: The Literature   30
Countering Those Slings and Arrows   34
Final Defense: Military Intelligence   35
Not-So-Dirty Tricks   36

Chapter 3. Hostilities Begin: The Announcement   39

The Paranoid Zone   40
How It Will Happen   41
When It Will Happen   43
What to Look For at the Announcement   43
Consultants   45
How to Tell Your Staff: Communication 101   47
The Library Staff As Tribe   49

Chapter 4. Phony War Syndrome (PWS)   **55**

Phony War Explained   55
Opportunities   58
Case Histories   58
Opportunities from Other Librarians   60
The Business Model   61
The Inner Circle and Positioning   62

Chapter 5. Planning Your Campaign   **67**

Trends in Libraries   68
Vision Statement   71
SWOT-ing Your Organization   73
Budgeting in a New Millennium   76
Consider Your Options   78

Chapter 6. The Big Presentation   **83**

Writing for Success   83
Powerful PowerPoint   85
Secrets of a Great Presentation   87
Case Histories   91
Conclusion   92

**Chapter 7. Implementing Your Battle Plans
and the Uh-Oh Factor**   **93**

Implementing Change   93
Outsourcing   95
Back to *Survivor*: The Merge   96
Retraining Staff   97
Layoffs: Beware the Executioner's Song   98
The Uh-Oh Factor and Backpedaling with Style   100
Conflict Resolution   102

Chapter 8. Surprise! You Are the One Downsized **105**

Benefits of Being Laid Off   106
The Severance Package: Negotiating the Best Deal   109
Fallacies of Downsizings   112
What to Do After You Have Been Laid Off   114

The Right Attitude   116
The Interview   117

Chapter 9. When Hostilities Cease   **121**

Aftermath   121
Alternatives to Downsizing   122
Survivor Syndrome   124
Dodos: A Cautionary Tale of the Future   126
Conclusion   133

Notes   **135**

Bibliography   **141**

Index   **149**

Preface

My one regret in life is that I am not someone else.

Woody Allen

This book started out detailing a health care–related phenomenon, the corporate downsizing, and other bad companywide events as they relate to medical librarians in their organization. Then the economics of the new millennium hit for-profit corporations, the public sector, and the education community. A sour economy was hit with the aftermath of 9/11 as surely and as cruelly as those airplanes hit the Twin Towers. Diminished revenues suddenly impacted the budgets in the public sector. Less tax revenue means less money for library services. For the first time, public librarians were confronted with budgetary issues they never had to confront before. The issues that turned my beard gray in the 1980s were being experienced by my friends and colleagues in all kinds of libraries in the new millennium. I found myself discussing and advising librarians from many different types of libraries.

Be prepared. Many times staff resign themselves to the negative events as they unfold. This will be shown to be the worst possible tactic. Stasis is akin to professional suicide. Don't dismiss this book or these issues as purely a part of the health care crisis. A downsizing may be coming to a library near you. It could be coming to your library. Consider this book as a cautionary tale. Ignore these lessons at your own risk.

This book is a true amalgam. I have taken research from the library literature, the hospital literature, business and finance, books on war and tactics (I am a former American History major, and make no mistake, in a downsizing, you will be in a battle zone), and the motivational literature.

A downsizing is first and foremost a business event, so the business literature was used extensively. If you were describing a hurricane, an event that devastates regardless of race, creed, or color similar to a downsizing, the meteorological literature would be invaluable. I mixed it all together with my personal experiences, interviews, and case histories. I have gone to my colleagues in the medical library community for their input. The research for this book would comprise three books the size of this one. It is a training manual for the librarians caught in the new millennium where shrinking budgets, inflated journal bills, and increasing demand for new expensive services are the order of the day.

Warning! Warning! Warning! This book contains opinions, not all of which are politically correct. It has adult content and language inappropriate for the fainthearted. It should have the print equivalent of a PG-13 rating. If you are offended by the terms B-school thugs, cold-blooded lizards, corporate dinosaurs, or mean-spirited administrative weasels, this book is not for you. The truth is not pretty (neither are most hospital executives). If you don't understand why Scott Adams makes fun of those nice administrative types in his terrible (wonderful) *Dilbert* comic strip, then this book is not for you. Experience does not always equate wisdom, but if you swim with sharks long enough, you become able to spot a dangerous fin from a distance or become fish food. I have swum with the sharks successfully for fifteen years and have the scars to prove it.

Acknowledgments

Recently I was given a very good review for my job performance at my place of employment for the preceding year, but the review had a caveat. Since there is no money for raises, it is strictly a symbolic review. I said, "It is not the award, as much as the honor of being nominated."

Just like the Academy Awards, this overstuffed pseudointellectual would like to acknowledge the contributions of the many people who made this book possible. My wife, Jan, always the commensurate editor, put up with a writer who would break all the rules for a laugh and threaten to burn the quiche if her editing was too vigorous. Without her toughness as a reporter and editor, this book would not have been possible. Many others helped. M. Sandra Wood, my editor at The Haworth Press, has been invaluable to me. She is a great editor and I listen to every constructive criticism she gently imparts. Many librarians assisted me with ideas including Amy Blaine, Leann Isaac, Elisabeth Jacobsen, Cleo Pappas, Titi Alexander, Maribeth Trost, and Marie Ferguson. All have proven the value of MEDLIB to me when I hit that infamous mental brick wall. A special thank you goes out to Lynn Sabol and Victoria Carlquist, two Connecticut librarians who are a credit to their profession. I feel honored to consider them my friends.

My colleagues at the West Virginia University, who interlibrary loaned articles for me, deserve special mention. They assisted me in locating a lot of great source material and consistently do a great job for their patrons.

To the famed mystery writers Marcia Talley and Lisa Scottoline, thank you for giving me encouragement at a time I really needed it. Ms. Talley's talk was inspirational.

To anyone I have missed, please forgive my omission. Many unsung heroes lent their support to my efforts with advice and great ideas and anecdotes.

Thank you all for believing in me more than I believed in myself.

Chapter 1

Introduction

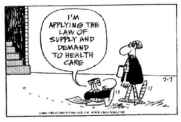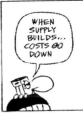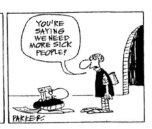

When the downsizing started at my hospital, I quipped, "When life gives you lemons make lemonade." By the end of the process, I was looking for limes to make margaritas.

Michael J. Schott

Once upon a time in the halcyon 1980s, a middle-management position in a hospital or university was a great job. Hospital salaries were good and raises were yearly. Librarians prepared their budgets for the next year by simply adding 10 percent to their previous budget. For younger librarians who did not have the pleasure of experiencing the 1980s and early 1990s in hospital library work, this is not a fairy tale. Journal inflation was low. If a librarian was fortunate enough to be at an academic institution, he or she was assured a position until retirement with a good pension. That was then. The boom years of the 1980s and early 1990s have given way to the bust years of the new millennium. The bubble burst. The paradigm shifted. Get over it.

Many library administrators intellectually reared during the boom years are unprepared for and are struggling with the bust. The literature is not helpful. Few articles have been written about the process of downsizing from a librarian's point of view. Only now have librarians begun to write about the frustrations and pain involved in this process. As more and more go through this process, librarians will start to tell their colleagues about their failures and successes as I did in my seminal article, "Corporate Downsizing and the Special Library (Getting Tired of Lemons)," which appeared in the *MLA News* in 1996.[1] Little did I know when I wrote that article that I was writing about the profession's future as much as my own past.

Librarians don't like downsizing. Their mission is to make order out of chaos. As a group, they don't like disorder. If you needed stuff put in the proper place so it could be retrieved later, whether it is books, videos, or Web sites, you would call on a librarian. Deep down in your heart, you know all your colleagues are suffering from obsessive-compulsive disorder and are candidates for heavy doses of Zoloft. You like to come in to work at the same time, and get your coffee or tea and sit down at your desk. You revel in the sameness of it all. You are not a chance taker. I learned very early in my library career not to move the stapler on another librarian's desk. The librarian animal thrives in a very organized environment and withers and dies in disorder.

What happens during a downsizing? Chaos reigns supreme. No matter what upper management's battle plan is, there is a great deal of uncertainty at this time. An old adage says that once you go into battle the plan gets thrown out. Your staff will bounce off the wall. All the order and sameness you had built into your life is suddenly swept away in a tide of change. You are going through a process that is totally opposed to your nature. Is it time you reassess your personal nature? Are you so opposed to change that you are in danger of becoming a career dinosaur?

The natural but dangerous tendency is to sweep bad news under the rug. One of the best parts of Tom Peters' *In Search of Excellence* (1985) video is when he talks about walking past the boss's blue-haired secretary, going into the big boss's office and saying, "Hey boss, let me tell you about the huge screwup that happened on the line today."[2] In real life, this scenario does not often happen. In these conservative times, no one easily admits failure. Failure is often too expensive. Scapegoats are immediately sought out. Americans prize success but don't take time to learn the lessons of failure.

Most library administration books written in kinder times paint a rosy picture of unlimited budgets for staff and operating expenses. Professors in library administration courses routinely assign projects to design libraries or expand preexisting libraries but never assign projects to contract libraries or deal with a downsizing. Why? Contraction is as much a fact of library administration as is expansion. Nothing adequately prepares the administrator for the bad times that are right around the corner.

A tendency these days is to say, "It's (the medical information) all on the Internet for free. Why do we need a library?" The Web is a powerfully competitive force. The all-on-the-Web argument is an extremely dangerous argument because it shows that the library director has not been doing his or her job of promoting the library to upper and middle management. If this argument is made, the director may have already lost the battle by not fielding an army. Sun Tzu in his *Art of War* states, "Thus it is that in war the victorious strategist only seeks battle after the victory has been won, whereas he who is destined to defeat first fights and afterwards looks for victory." If enough people think a department is superfluous, it is superfluous. Perception rules when the cost-cutting mob is in charge, and make no mistake about it being a mob. It can be a raucous, out-of-control mob that makes the French Revolution look like a walk in the park. You may be the one pushing the cart to the guillotine or you may be in the cart. Everyone gets to play. There are no time-outs.

Upper management can separate itself from the bloodletting by assigning the "dirty work" to middle-management teams led by outside consultants. It may be a library manager's colleagues who do the cutting. It may be you. You will make the plans, implement them, and take the heat if they fail. You may be the executioner. You will counsel the ones who are laid off and the dysfunctional survivors who remain, full of anger, frustration, and shock. You will explain to your friends who you have worked with for years why they are suddenly not needed by the organization, knowing that their families will bear the brunt of the devastation your actions have caused. You were only following orders. You will pick up the pieces. For many library managers, this will be their first time making these kinds of decisions.

One director said to me, "I have always hired. I have never had to fire anyone in twenty years as a director."

CORPORATE VIEW OF DOWNSIZING

Most hospitals are corporations, which means they are limited liability financial and legal entities set up in a certain way to meet certain federal regulations.[3] Whether they are not-for-profit or for-profit corporations does not matter. What walks like a duck is usually a duck and anyone who has ever attended a morning report knows that young doctors should never go looking for zebras when they hear hoof-beats. It is important to understand the nature of corporations before discussing health care.

First, one must believe that corporations are living, breathing organisms with a vested interest in their own survival. Sometimes the organism is capable of incredible evil in its struggle for survival. For-profit corporations must make a profit for their shareholders. Without shareholder confidence and investment, there is no new funding for expansion. Not-for-profit corporations must break even, have funds for raises and expansion and support their philanthropic endeavors.

Corporations downsize to prune an ineffective bureaucracy, lower overhead costs, shorten the decision-making process, and thus better respond to market forces, improve communication in the organization, and improve productivity.[4] They expand and grow in good times and contract in bad. They make poor decisions or the market changes. They fail to adequately deal with the change. Some become obsolete as their goods and services are no longer needed. You can think of buggy whip manufacturers at the beginning of the twentieth century. They experienced a dramatic downsizing as their products were no longer needed.

A surprising fact is that not only corporations in trouble downsize. Most employees have a misconception that if their company is doing well, their jobs are secure. Studies have shown that healthy companies downsize to reduce costs and boost earnings by reducing headcount.[5] These corporations also try to preempt hard times instead of reacting to them. This cutting when cutting is not needed has a backlash effect. Employees become extremely jaded and have no loyalty to their employers as their employers show them no loyalty.

Corporations look upon downsizing as a natural process that is necessary for the continued health of the organization. Sometimes there is fat that must be cut away. Corporations also consider downsizing part of the change process. Change happens. Good corporations recognize change and deal with it. We will discuss change later on in this chapter.

Regrettably, some corporations see their employees as valuable assets but in a negative way. As Dilbert might say, they fire a few of them and their stock goes up. In some of the organizations in which I have worked, Dilbert was worshiped as a god.

PARADIGM SHIFT WITHOUT A CLUTCH

Sometimes the most profound things are the simplest. Things change. This is a very small idea but a very profound one. You do not cook food the way your parents did (if you own a microwave). If you have a cell phone, you do not communicate the same as your parents did. You use a computer—a relatively new invention. You probably own a VCR, DVD, and a CD player. (It took the DVD only six years to pass videotape in sales and rentals). Major social and technological changes are happening all around you. Do you recognize them? More important, can you recognize the real shifts, adapt, and profit from them?

In 1962, Thomas Kuhn wrote *The Structure of Scientific Revolution*. He coined the phrase "paradigm shift." A paradigm shift can be defined as a change from one way of thinking (and doing things) to another.[6] It does not just happen. It is driven by the agents of change. Usually the new way is superior to the old way and people take up the banner of the new.

Alvin Toffler, in his groundbreaking book *Future Shock,* tells of how change is speeding up. For centuries people relied on the same knowledge. During the Middles Ages, how a man farmed was how his father or grandfather farmed.[7] Johannes Gutenberg's invention of the printing press started a revolution that is continuing today. Change is accelerating at an alarming rate. We must all adapt to CDs then DVDs then whatever comes next. Have you noticed that the twenty-fourth-century toys of *Star Trek*-like cell phones are appearing in the twenty-first century? As a culture, our technology is outdistancing our ability to imagine the future. The twenty-fourth century is tomorrow.

A lesson in paradigm shifts comes from the Swiss watch industry. At one time almost all quality watches were manufactured in Switzerland. Then the cheap digital watches came along in the 1970s, changing people's perceptions of watches. The Swiss did not understand or recognize this change and their watch industry nearly went out of business.

What does this mean to library administrators? We must be mindful of change. Yesterday there were card catalogs. Then came electronic catalogs. Then Web-based catalogs appeared. Recognize change before it happens. Plan for it and deal with it before it becomes a reality. A good manager wonders, "What is coming next? How can I prepare for this new reality?"

The electronic card catalog spawned copy cataloging that impacted forever the catalogers' jobs in libraries. Will full-text online databases do the same for the interlibrary loan librarian? If everything is online have we leapfrogged the need for this position? Should we take the resources from one area and apply them to the new one? If librarians don't make these decisions they will become the buggy whip makers of the new millennia.

HEALTH CARE REALITY

In health care, the federal Medicare budget cuts that began in the 1980s had much to do with the present poor state of affairs.[8] So hospitals in the late 1980s did what for-profit corporations had already done: they countered reduced revenues by reducing expenses. Namely, they reduced staff. The B-school mentality had taken over health care (it is no small coincidence that downsizing followed the invasion of health care by the B-school clones). It has been noted that many B-schools teach that employees are expenses to be minimized, not assets to be maximized. Good corporations treat their employees as valuable capital in whom they have invested heavily.

Hospitals that relied on Medicare for their revenues were hit very hard, sending them into a tailspin. Then came the Balanced Budget Act of 1997, which further reduced Medicare payments.[9] Hospitals are still spiraling downward. Although businesses, hospitals are unique in that they must treat all who arrive at their doors regardless of ability to pay. They assume billions of dollars in debt each year from unpaid bills. More and more the uninsured are not the underclass but the middle class as corporations cut back on coverage. Hospitals in border states are going bankrupt treating illegal aliens without health insurance. Medicare pays about 60 percent of a hospital bill. Many times the hospital must assume responsibility for the other 40 percent. What corporation could survive if it got less than 60 percent of list price for its goods or services?

Medical technology is another issue. Equipment ages or is replaced at an alarming rate in today's high-tech world. Could this be the Toffler effect of accelerated change in action? New developments make old procedures and tests obsolete, but new procedures are more expensive. Hospitals must bear the brunt of constant equipment and computer upgrades. Along with this, because of advanced medical technology, many medical procedures that were inpatient only are now outpatient procedures. I recently read an article on the possibility of making heart surgery an outpatient procedure. Once a miracle of science, soon a cardiac catheterization may be a very mundane event performed as an outpatient.

Censuses are drastically down at hospitals all over the country and a general discussion is going on about too many empty hospital beds in U.S. hospitals. From 1988 to 1994, there was an excess of nearly 1,000 beds in many major cities. By 1998 that excess was estimated to soar to 3,000 to 4,000 beds.[10]

After the budgetary disasters of the late 1980s, many hospitals went into the rehabilitation services business in which the reimbursement was still good. Common wisdom was that managed care and the government wanted patients out of the hospital as quickly as possible, into rehabilitation facilities, and back to work. So rehabilitation facilities became the rage with hospitals. The Balanced Budget Act of 1997 closed that loophole by cutting reimbursement for nursing home facilities, leaving hospitals with diminished incomes from off-site facilities.[11] This seems counterproductive to the idea of releasing people from the hospital as quickly as possible and it cut off an important profit center for hospitals.

Several medical ethical issues should be addressed. Malpractice confronts and confounds health care. Insurance rates have increased at an alarming rate due in part to the downturn in the economy and the subsequent loss of insurance companies' investments in the stock market. Hospitals have been forced to pick up some of the cost of malpractice insurance or lose good doctors in critical specialties such as orthopedic surgery.

Issues concerning end-of-life treatment and the high cost of drugs make health care a volatile arena. America seems unable to resolve the medical ethics issues that plague and bleed it dry such as end-of-life support or substance abuse treatment. Lack of a consensus on these issues has hamstrung timid politicians.

Managed care companies sprung up in the 1990s to deal with out of control health care costs. They have helped to get the best price for their members, but they are siphoning money out of the health care system with overall mixed results. After fifteen years of health maintenance organizations limiting access to health care, it does not seem as if America is any healthier or costs any better. How much health care costs are actually kept down is debatable.

Some counter that a universal health care system would solve these woes. Think again. Although I toured a British hospital and have nothing but respect for their system, the Canadian universal health care system, similar to the British system, has been in financial trouble since the 1980s. They have had their own rounds of drastic downsizings and the trend does not appear to have abated. Between 1986-1987 and 1994-1995 the number of public hospitals in Canada fell by 14 percent and the number of approved beds in these hospitals declined by 11 percent.[12]

Hospital libraries have their own unique problems. In 1983, the Department of Human Services eliminated the maintenance of hospital libraries as a qualification for reimbursement for Medicare and Medicaid.[13] This short-sighted edict kicked one of the most important supports out from under the hospital library. Subsequent weakening of JCAHO (Joint Commission on Accreditation of Healthcare Organizations) standards left the hospital library teetering as precariously as a clown on a three-legged stool balancing on just one leg. The hushed audience waits with bated breath for the clown to come crashing down.

Nonmedical librarians and library school students may be reading this and think hospitals are full of danger and disagreeable people, and are horrible places for librarians. This is not true for many of us. Hospitals can be very exciting places where what you do saves people's lives. Physicians have told me point blank that my efforts changed how they treated a patient. No job I have had has ever been as intense or as rewarding as working in a hospital. Nothing compares with the rush of that first search when "the patient is going south," but there is considerable heat in working in a hospital environment in which lives are on the line. Tempers flair and huge egos can ruin your day. Exhausted physicians are not happy to get bills for overdue interlibrary loans or books. As the old saying goes, "If you can't stand the heat . . ." Heat can be both beneficial and dangerous to the wielder.

FIGURES DON'T LIE, LIARS FIGURE

If you are an American worker, chances are you will be involved in some way in a downsizing during the course of your working life. It has been estimated that over 43 million jobs have vanished since 1979. Nearly three-quarters of all households have had a close encounter with a downsizing since 1980. In one-third of all households a family member has lost a job. Nearly 40 percent know a friend, relative, or neighbor who has lost a job.[14] Automation is partly to blame; our technology is replacing its makers. Few realized how many middle-management jobs would die when computers came into the workplace. Fewer realized that NAFTA (North American Free Trade Agreement) would send so many middle-management jobs offshore. The spreadsheet has replaced the bookkeeper. The middle manager is now expendable.

In 1984, the largest 500 companies in the United States employed more than 14 million people. In 1994, those same companies employed less than 12 million.[15] In 1993, 27 percent of 1,147 hospitals surveyed planned to decrease their staff in the next year. That same year, 35 percent of the vice presidents of nursing in North Carolina hospitals reported a downsizing in the past three years.[16] That was at the end of the first wave of downsizings that began in the late 1980s.

In another survey of hospital CEOs, it was reported that 57 percent of those polled said that their hospital had in the past five years implemented a hospital-wide reengineering.[17] In the current era, a new round of deep cuts has occurred. It was estimated that between 1995 and 1997, 750,000 new jobs would be lost in health care.[18] In 2001, only eighty-three mergers occurred. It seems a small number, unless your hospital was one of the hospitals merged.

While researching downsizing for this book, I came across an article written in 1993 stating that most hospital downsizing would occur at the upper-management level because that is where the big salaries are and where the fat is. A whole level of upper management would be eliminated at some hospitals and middle managers would do the work of upper management. The few upper-administrative types left would support middle managers—the ones who actually do the work.[19] Looking back, the article was unintentionally hilarious and one of the best pieces of inadvertent social satire that I have ever read.

DEFINITIONS

As a medical librarian and manager in a hospital, university, or corporate entity, many bad things can happen (referred to in this book as a bad corporate event [BCE]). In fact, hundreds of methods and scenarios exist in which one may lose funding but the end result is that a librarian has to do more with less. This is an oxymoron on the level with jumbo shrimp or military intelligence. It is also what good-managing medical librarians deal with daily.

This book deals with the extremely bad things that can happen to a medical librarian to ruin his or her day. The following is a list of some BCEs:

- *Across-the-board budget cut.* Who said, "The first cut is the deepest?" Rod Stewart, Cat Stevens, the hospital librarian, or Hannibal Lecter? (The correct answer is all of the above.) This is where one gives back a portion of one's budget. Since the average library's budget has two major line items—staff and printed materials—the choices are few. Typically these cuts are announced at the worst possible time, such as right after you have sent in that approved journal list to your vendor. Whether the money will be there next year is irrelevant: it is gone and the smart manager must manage differently than he or she did when the money was there. In some organizations this is done yearly and staff know to spend all their money by a certain date before they must give it back. Some library managers try to manage as if the cut didn't happen, thus ignoring a paradigm shift in the very worse way. Paradigm shifts are all about reality. Ignore reality at your own risk. Less means less. Ultimately, the yearly midyear budget cut becomes a cynical process in which the department head asks for more money than necessary based on the annual midseason giveback. In fact, in this process everyone lies. The administrator gives you a budget knowing full well he or she is going to take it back. The library director takes the money and spends as much as he or she can before the cutoff point.

- *Downsizing (also called dumbsizing or rightsizing).* Downsizing reduces the number of employees on the operating payroll permanently. A target number or percentage is usually involved. Please note, nonrevenue-generating departments (support staff) are many times the first to be cut.

- *Stealth downsizing.* This is a particular favorite of mine. The manager comes into work one day and finds that a particular class of manager or vice president has been eliminated. In a newspaper interview a retiring painter at a hospital spoke of how he hated to do a renovation of an office in the afternoon because the administrator would come back from lunch not knowing why the painter was removing the administrator's nameplate from the door. The painter was left to explain to the administrator that he or she had been fired. He hated doing that.

- *Reorganization or reengineering (also called a restructuring).* This is the fundamental rethinking and radical redesign of business processes to achieve dramatic improvements in critical, contemporary measures of performance, such as cost, quality, service, and speed. This involves a restructuring of the entire organization. Unlike a downsizing that is geared to eliminate staff, the economies in a reengineering eliminate waste through process change. Many times, departments are combined for efficiency. The objectives are to achieve higher levels of labor productivity, thus enabling hospitals to deliver care at lower costs without adversely affecting patient satisfaction and quality of care. Think of it as a downsizing with expensive suits (consultants). After a while, staff get gun-shy and start to recognize the expensive suits going into administrative offices. The rumors go through the organization like wildfire. In the history of the known world there has probably never been a reorganization during which staff have been added. An old soldiers' saying states, "We've got too many troops in this room." I like to end my lecture on downsizing by posing a scenario: "You are called into the auditorium with all the other managers in the hospital. You are separated into groups of ten. Each group of ten managers goes into a separate room. They are given orders that only eight can come out with jobs. What would you do?" Seldom do I get a good answer.

- *Buyout or severance package.* Anyone in the organization with a certain amount of accrued pension time may be eligible for an early pension package. It's a buyout of the expensive senior employees. It is like getting a "get out of jail free card" in Monopoly. The problem is you have little or no control over who leaves and who stays. What would you do if your best, most experienced, and well-trained employees suddenly vanished, leaving you without the employee resources to complete your department's mission? In one buyout, I lost 40 percent of my staff. Are a large number of your staff close to retirement age? What is your plan? Cross-training, anyone?
- *Merger.* This procedure combines two or more entities into one, through a purchase or a pooling of interests. It differs from a consolidation in that no new entity is created from a merger. Usually one hospital consumes or merges with the other. The rationale for a merger is economies of scale. If two separate libraries exist, there may be an impetus to reduce or eliminate one. Which one? Seldom does one hear a librarian say, "Take me, take me."
- *Consolidation.* The combining of separate companies, functional areas, or product lines, into a single one. It differs from a merger in that a new entity is created in the consolidation.

None of these problems is in the least bit enjoyable for a manager. As a matter of fact, the emotional issues raised by these problems are an important part of this book. Enormous emotional collateral damage is caused by every decision a library manager makes during this process. The collateral damage is suffered by the cutter as much as the cuttee. Like war, there are no winners. If a library manager understands this, it may save him or her many trips to the therapist and minimize the collateral damage to staff. It is easy to win a Pyrrhic victory. One wins the battle but at such a high price he or she ultimately loses the war. The emotional damage can be so great that the staff never recover. Studies show that many disillusioned and depressed staff leave a hospital after a downsizing. Each of these scenarios is fraught with difficulties. Each has its own set of traps for the library manager. Successfully negotiating the minefields, maintaining services, and recognizing and dealing with new paradigms is why the library manager gets the big bucks (at least that is what the staff who earn less think). But management is all about making hard decisions. Real managers make hard decisions in bad times. Real managers survive and thrive even in bad times.

This book will work through the typical scenario of a downsizing, budget cut, merger, or pension buyout. Such events follow a pattern. If you know the pattern you can understand what is going on and deal with it. Most parents who go through Lamaze class have seen that videotape of ten births. The theory is that after watching ten couples go through the trials and joys of birth, you will accept it for the natural beautiful thing it is and go with the flow. You will be desensitized to the process and better able to handle it. Welcome to the birthing of a BCE with all the pain and agony of the real thing. It comes out ripping and slashing. I cannot guarantee that your BCE will exactly follow this guide. Maybe there won't be a corporatewide announcement. Maybe there will not be a phony war period. It is guaranteed that some of what you are going to experience has already been experienced and can be documented. Thus defined, it can be studied and dealt with. Pick the elements you need this time and discard the rest. The book is chock-full of advice from battle-scarred veterans of the downsizing wars.

You are about to enter a dimension not of sight and sound but of mind—a place where chaos reigns and nothing is as it seems. Your colleagues may remain your friends or suddenly become your worst enemies. When everyone is trying to grasp at a single life preserver some people drown. Sometimes, while you are grasping the life preserver, you may watch someone you know or care about drown and feel great guilt that you are a survivor.

THE NASTIEST SECRET OF ALL

Caught up in the pain and emotional trauma, you may not realize that the downsizing or reengineering in your hospital has failed. A large number of downsizings do not succeed. Bet they don't tell you that at the first announcement.

It is estimated that two-thirds of reengineering projects fail or fall significantly short of their hoped-for outcomes. Less than 33 percent of the corporations surveyed met their profit objectives the first year after a downsizing.[20] There may be resistance to change in the organization, unrealistic expectations, or lack of a clear purpose or goal. Sometimes managers and administration just go through the motions. All such occurrences can doom a downsizing.

Regrettably, downsized employees may impact the hospital's ability to bounce back when good times return. Without adequate staff to handle new business, the organization cannot grow.

The worst secret of all is that one downsizing may lead to a whole series of downsizings in your organization. You have heard of serial killings? Consider a serial downsizing during which the fun never ends.

Good upper management realizes that their downsizing has failed and amends those mistakes. They realize they are paying outside contractors more than they paid their former employees for the same services. Good upper management is flexible enough to make amends. Don't be surprised if the colleague you bid good-bye to with a dinner and a tearful hug is suddenly back at his or her old job, occasionally with a raise. During one downsizing I participated in, 25 percent of the downsized staff were hired back—some as consultants. There may be an opportunity to get your staff back. Can you recognize that opportunity and take advantage of it? What elements do you look for to tell if the downsizing will work (based on the announcement) or is working? What do you do if it doesn't work? What will the downsizing mean to your career?

As in war, acts of great heroism and great cowardice occur. During one downsizing I turned to a person that I had a ten-year running battle with and said, "Being on this committee, I realize for the first time your incredible talents as a conciliator. Many times you have saved this process and me by keeping a cool head. I have watched you work harder than anyone to make this process work. I think you are a wonderful team leader and facilitator." In the blink of an eye, the conflict of ten years was washed away and that person became a good friend.

In this book, I will detail some of the incredible acts of absurdity I have witnessed. One hospital I worked at responded to a drop in revenues by eliminating ketchup packets from the cafeteria condiment tray. This did little to stem the bleeding caused by increases in suppliers' prices, unprofitable divisions, or competitors stealing market share. Remarkably, the "ketchup packet affair" earned management considerable bad will with line employees that took years to overcome. Ten years later, people were still referring to it as a mean-spirited decision by management. Having gone through this process a number of times, I can relate some experiences that may be invaluable to the novice. People do bizarre things under stress.

The stakes are small, just your career and family's lifestyle in these great United States. If you survive, you and your work will be forever changed, and not always for the better. You are about to enter The Downsizing Zone. Like Dante's *Inferno,* the sign over the door should read, "Abandon all hope, ye who enter here."

Chapter 2

Arming Yourself
(Before the Announcement)

I can feel it coming in the air tonight.

Phil Collins

Even paranoids have real enemies.

Henry Kissinger

Will the real enemies in the room raise their hands?

Michael J. Schott

I like to use another saying that goes, "Before engaging in a battle of wits, one must ensure that one's opponent is armed." Are you armed? You are about to go into battle against the fiercest fire-breathing dragon in the forest. Many librarians go off with only their own self-righteousness as defense and get toasted. (Self-righteousness makes poor armor.) Your livelihood, your staff, your professional reputation, and your family's happiness and mental health are all at stake. Better carry something into that fight besides your preconceptions and worn catchphrases from *Library Journal*.

One of the difficulties with being a corporate librarian is that unlike your public library brethren who tend to congregate in protective groups, you may be a single librarian in a large corporate entity standing alone and exposed. Not everyone speaks your language or has your values. Others in your company or hospital may not believe in the book as a penultimate medium of information or that hospitals need libraries. Marketing in this environment is a constant job as new "uneducated" staff come on board all the time. A good orientation program is vital to help newbies understand the uses and need for a corporate library. Remember, according to the powers that be, all the information is on the Web anyway. Know your enemy and go into battle well prepared and properly armed.

SECRET ARROW IN THE QUIVER:
THE RÉSUMÉ

Okay, first, go to your desk, fire up your computer, and access your résumé. Battles are seldom won by conflicted warriors. Your personal house must be in order before you are ready to do battle. During the downsizing process, a time may come when you as a manager may decide that the emotional or moral cost is too high. Some of the decisions you make may be in that gray area that Scott Adams likes to refer to as the "way of the weasel," where not completely moral decisions are made—the "Bill was out sick today and couldn't be here so our committee will cut him and tell him about it later" kind of decisions. I still remember the time in seventh grade when I was out sick with the flu, and upon returning to school I found out that I had been made Tiny Tim in the school Christmas play. Weasels live in elementary schools just as surreally as they live in corporations. (Where do corporate weasels come from—corporate weasel schools?) After three performances and saying "God bless us everyone" in front of the entire school, I was never out sick for the remainder of the school year.

You may hear about horror stories from other hospitals that have gone through the process. If they use the same consultants, you can expect the same treatment. You may get wind that your hospital is planning on merging with another larger hospital and your entire department is on the chopping block. You see a job advertised on a local job board. The job may have better pay or a better commute. Maybe it is more secure. You seriously consider applying. There is nothing ignoble about skipping the process entirely and killing yourself off. In some cases librarians have successfully migrated to other jobs during this process and saved themselves a great deal of grief (downsized themselves). One librarian director told me, "I solved our downsizing problem and got a better job. I downsized myself." The reality is that he probably saved his organization about $90,000 by resigning when it takes more than a year to recruit a new person for the position he left. He needed to cut about $90,000 to cover his shortfall. Downsizing can be a painful process. It is a process during which, to borrow a phrase from Comrade Khrushchev describing a nuclear exchange, "The living will envy the dead." Sometimes it is better to be dead and gone. Sometimes the survivors envy the ones who are gone.

When was the last time you updated your résumé? When you accepted your present job? This leaves you very vulnerable. Never wait until you need your résumé. We all enter the downsizing process thinking we are far too valuable to the organization to be laid off. Mistakes happen. One thing you will learn is that the wrong people are cut during downsizings. You could be the one let go. Like a necessary machine, your résumé should be cared for and well-oiled. Think of it as your vehicle in need of a 3,000-mile oil change and tune up your résumé monthly. Things happen very quickly in this job market. Be ready; have an escape plan.

The librarian résumé is a strange bird. Today the average librarian is part academic, part literature researcher, part civil servant, part help desk guru, part administrator, and part computer techie. The good résumé should reflect all of these elements. Look at your résumé. Have you included your present position? Why not? Aren't you doing things that reflect value and would be valuable to a new employer?

What do you do? Have you learned new skills? Have you remodeled the facilities? Installed new systems? Trained staff or patrons in the use of databases or software? Have you written any manuals? Written a new Web page? Won any awards? Have you written any articles that have appeared in peer-reviewed journals? Given any lectures at statewide or national conferences? Served on any professional committees? Pioneered the use of new technology? Are you proud of something you do? What are you good at? Transmit this enthusiasm to your résumé, then wait for the interviews.

Is your résumé a list of job descriptions from your past jobs and not a list of your achievements on those jobs?[1] Are there any significant employment gaps that should be explained? Have you job-hopped before? Most employees in America stay at a job for two to three years. If you have had many jobs in a short period, this should be addressed, as it is a major red flag with prospective employers.

Some résumés are too honest. They detail every flaw or problem with their former places of employment. They describe in detail why the person was laid off. This is not necessary. It is perfectly okay to just say the positive things that you did at your last job and eliminate the negative. You can cover these points during the interview. (The interview is discussed in Chapter 8.)

It is recommended that you think of your targeted résumé and why your prospective employer would consider you a successful candidate. What key elements would you bring to the position that would ensure your success?[2] Employers don't want to fire and re-interview. It takes time and is expensive. If they see a great candidate with a good chance of success, they will bite. Remember, an employer in the corporate setting may view your résumé for an average of eight seconds on the initial pass. You have eight seconds to make a lasting impression with that prospective employer.

This is the time for you to brag about yourself. Make the most of it. Any important thing that you have done should be on your résumé. It is the only communication between that prospective employer and you. Make it a good one. And spell-check that document. Many jobs have been lost because of a sloppy résumé. Have someone who is not a librarian look it over to remove the jargon. Clarity is very important. Invest in some good paper to print the résumé on. Don't put a great résumé (career) that you are proud of on poor-quality paper. You are worth more than that.

POSITIVE POWER OF GREAT LEADERSHIP

Much has been written about the "L" word. Everyone has an opinion on the issue of leadership. Recent studies show that a very important part of leadership is attitude. You cannot change many things. You cannot change your staff. They need their paychecks and don't want to lose pension benefits by moving to another job. You cannot significantly change your funding. It will be the same because that is how the organization perceives your department's value. However, you *can* change your attitude.[3]

Studies show that a mark of a successful leader is his or her positive attitude. This may seem like a no-brainer to a lot of people. Some may quote famous tough bosses as exceptions that negate this rule. Still, when all is said and done, your mood translates down to your staff. If you are negative, your staff may be negative. In a customer-focused organization, negative staff can be disastrous. Comments such as "that is not my job" or "that is a stupid request" can doom you. Negative staff will not take healthy risks. Why take risks when you are just going to fail? Negative staff do not share vital information among themselves or with you. Fear and anxiety are prevalent in a negative staff culture. Tense or terrified staff are not productive.

Your emotional mood is vital to the health of your organization. Scientists have found that the more you act negatively in your workplace, the more it is ingrained in your brain circuitry.[4] We create a never-ending loop reinforcing these feelings. Then our staff pick up on these feelings, and they are transmitted through the entire organization. If you snap at people when you are stressed or angry (and it is okay to be angry), what will your staff do when they are mad or stressed? What do your children do when they see you do something wrong?

Know what is going on in your organization. Keep the lines of communication open. Listen to staff when they talk to you. You don't have to institute a 360-degree feedback program but don't turn away from constructive criticism. When you know what is going on, you can self-manage. Leave the bad feelings out of the office and deal with problems in an objective manner. Then, communicate your intentions to your staff clearly and convincingly, disarming conflicts.

Your staff will respond to this type of honest leadership. They will be happier. They will make you proud and protect your back. Good feelings will generate good feelings. One final thing should be mentioned about positive attitude. Just like your résumé, your attitude needs to be in top shape before a downsizing. You are in for a very rocky ride. You will have to rely on yourself to survive. Do what you must do with panache. Your attitude is not the only important aspect of leadership, and it is never a substitute for inaction. But it can be the spark that ignites great things in your organization.

SWORD IN THE SCABBARD: THE MISSION STATEMENT

If you do not have a clear, well-written mission statement for your library or have not reviewed your mission statement in the past year, you are jumping out of an airplane without a parachute. Your painful landing will be similar in both cases. (It's not the fall that will kill you but the abrupt stop.) You do not have the option of picking up a tape recorder hidden in a park bench at an out-of-the-way location, punching the play button and hearing, "Good morning, Ms. Phelps, your mission, should you choose to accept it, is . . ." Ah, for that kind of clarity in life. You also cannot use the phrase (when asked what your mission is), "To boldly go where no one has gone before." It's been done. I have used that phrase several times in executive correspondence. Regrettably, upper management did not understand the cultural reference (and they say librarians are humorless).

A good mission statement defends you like a sharp, broad sword. If you have a corporate-sanctioned mission, you have tacit corporate approval. Without it, you are just another extraneous department. A good mission statement expresses a department's reason for being; it conveys the department's identity and articulates purpose. It is simple stability in a world of change.

A good mission statement contains several basic elements. A mission statement is written to an audience and for an audience. Before writing the statement, a library manager must decide who his or her primary customers are. You must know your target audience.[5] If there are many divergent audiences, more than one statement could be in order.

A good mission statement is succinct and it should be no longer than thirty to forty words.[6] Try describing what you do in less than a hundred words. A mission statement should make a haiku seem like a Russian novel. It is very difficult to be as clear and brief as a good mission statement demands. Expect to write many drafts as you hone down your thoughts. If your human resources department is helpful, contact them for assistance in writing your mission statement.

Your mission statement should have the proper tone. If the language is too lofty or too humorous, it may have a negative effect on your audience and transmit the wrong message. Your mission statement should avoid bombast and state achievable goals. Biting off more than you can chew leaves patrons just as disappointed as not doing enough.

Try to factor in or write in a way to measure your mission statement's goals. If you have generalized pie-in-the-sky aspirations, how do you know you are achieving them? There is something to be said for the *Star Trek* approach: "To boldly go where no one has gone before." A good mission statement has stretch goals. You are always working harder to do more. This may seem like a contradiction of the previous statement about not disappointing patrons, but you, as a manager, must make those decisions and walk that fine line.

A mission statement should not be done as part of a SWOT (strengths, weaknesses, opportunities, threats) analysis.[7] We will save the organization SWOT-ing for later. A mission statement should be written after a great deal of strategic planning. Where should the library be in five years? How can we get to that place? What equipment will we need? What talents are we lacking? Is our staff the right mix of skills to achieve these goals? What organizations in the hospital will be needed to achieve our goals? These are a few questions that should be answered.

I can give one recommendation from experience. Advice from other managers can be politically motivated and thus dangerous. Beware of other managers' agendas. Managers are supposed to go into this process with the corporation's best interests at heart. This is seldom the case. Five managers may come into the room with ten different agendas. Saving their best friends from layoffs and acquiring new departments under their wing are only two of the motives you need to watch out for. I once had to fight off acquisition by another department. The department head tried to assume control by rewriting the library's mission statement to make the interloper the library's only customer. Only you know what your library should be doing. This is not a time for group thought or frivolous advice, although input from stakeholders may be important.

Once the statement is written then you can get the rest of the staff to buy in. A mission statement creates unity in an organization and a sense of purpose. When asked, staff can repeat the mission statement and be guided by it. Many times in libraries, support staff must act with initiative to satisfy an unusual request for information. Whether your organization succeeds or fails may rest on how the staff interprets the mission statement.

When the statement is written, it should be approved by the highest corporate entity. Preferably, it should be at the board level. Getting the library before the board should be something to work for. Do you read all board minutes, find out what interests the board members have, and try to send them information based on their interests? It is never a bad idea to have friends on the board.

As with your résumé (and you can consider your mission statement your corporate résumé), a mission statement is a work in progress. It should be taken out, dusted off, and revised when necessary at least once a year before you plan your corporate goals for the year.

When your colleagues want to cut the library to shreds, a board-approved mission statement is a very good thing to have.

MACE OF RIGHTEOUS:
YOUR MANAGEMENT STYLE

How well do you manage? This can be a scary question, but good management staves off the "slings and arrows of outrageous fortune." The following are some bits of advice from an expert in small-business management. You should:

- *Be inclusive.* With a small staff in which everyone plays a vital role, it is important that everyone feel equal and involved.[8] This includes those night staff people that you don't often see.
- *An effective boss establishes a genuine mission.* Not only can a clear mission serve to rally the troops, it can infuse employees with a sense of importance in their jobs. Your employees shouldn't fear the reaper. This is another concept that has been briefly mentioned before. Staff should not be afraid to experiment or try something new.[9]
- *Lead and don't forget to coach.* Coaching involves totally different skills than leading. You have to learn to support your staff. Compliment them. Make changes when necessary. See the whole field.
- *Help others' careers, too.* Some of us are very good at managing our own careers but fail to realize that staff have aspirations too. This is tricky business. You can assist good staff right out of the building if you are not careful. On the other hand, you can get the reputation as a great mentor and a stepping-stone for capable people.
- *Great bosses are made, not born. Leadership skills are acquired traits.*[10] We don't know how to lead when we are born. Try every day to improve your skills. Read management texts. Take any courses your hospital offers. Get a mentor. Use what you have. If you are a good parent, perhaps you can transfer these skills to your management style. If you are a good writer, memos and supportive literature may be your way to motivate. You have traits you don't realize you have. Accept criticism and do better next time.

STOUT SHIELD OF THE ARM:
CERTIFICATIONS AND REGULATIONS

I believe in the various certifications and regulations that make a library a necessary part of a hospital. I harken back to the fine hospital librarians in Connecticut during my tenure there, who realized that their greatest defense is the statutes.

In 1987, the Connecticut State Medical Society adopted the Medical Library Association's "Minimum Standards for Health Sciences Libraries" due to lobbying by the state medical librarians. In 1990, a medical librarian was added to every Connecticut Medical Society team that inspected hospitals for certification for the hospital to grant continuing medical education credits (CMEs).

Every three years, one of these inspection teams, made up of an administrator, a physician, and a librarian, goes to every hospital in the state to check and see if their policies are adequate, their facilities are adequate, and their staff are adequate for teaching purposes. A medical librarian inspects the library to see if it is adequate for medical residents or physicians based on standards approved by the state hospital library association and the state medical society. Most inspection teams treat the librarian as a full member of the team, and thus he or she not only rules on such matters as numbers of books but on outside sponsorship of educational opportunities.[11]

Librarians should aspire to this level and type of duties in every health care organization. If a hospital does not meet standards, it is cited. Too many cites and it may lose its accreditation and ability to grant CMEs. This would be a significant blow to the hospital's prestige and ability to recruit new physicians. On this committee, medical librarians have clout.

This was a brilliant move by the medical librarians in Connecticut. They have used their "big stick" many times to convince hospitals to improve library facilities and to keep librarians in the smallest of hospitals. It has given the librarians in the state a great deal of status in their organizations as well as statewide.

If you are not familiar with the physician groups in your county and state, address this issue now. Some of your best friends and biggest supporters are the physicians who work in your hospital. They will fight for you if given half the chance. They are a great source of local grants. Know and work with the director of continuing medical education in your hospital. Get on the speaker's bureau for your hospital and do a lecture at physician functions. See how many representatives of the state medical society are in your hospital and work with them.

Offer to help them with any state medical society projects they may be working on. Get in touch with the state hospital association. Find out if it has a librarian and go visit. Most librarians would deny the hospital librarian's political role. We are all politicians. We must be able to build consensus. We bring business into our organizations based on our personal styles.

One thing you can do to build consensus is to lecture at the local medical society on a topic such as MEDLINE or search engines. Make friends. Community physicians can be a resource. They are sometimes desperately isolated and would love help with research in this era of constant malpractice suits. Before you go to the meeting, do a little research and find out what information issues are hot buttons and talk about how you can help the physicians with those problems.

Review the IRB (institutional review board) standards for your library and the MLA (Medical Library Association) Standards for Hospital Libraries. They have specific recommendations for the size and scope of library services for certain size hospitals, going as far as making staffing and physical plant recommendations. Your colleagues worked long and hard to make those standards the best they can be. The MLA definitions of knowledge-based services mesh well with the definitions in the JCAHO manual.

Find out who in your organization is on the joint commission team in your hospital. The standards for the joint commission have been watered down over the years, but it is still good to review them now and then. Likewise, if your hospital has medical residents, then their programs must be inspected by the board for that specialty. An inspection of the library is usually a part of the hospital inspection. It is a very good idea to know when the inspections are to take place so you can correct any deficiencies before they become citations. Send a list of just-purchased books to the program director so he or she has them when the site inspector asks. Understand the library and information requirements of each residency. Go to the residency chairman and ask for the library requirement for that particular specialty. Keep a file on the specialty requirements. If you are not on the education committee at your hospital, ask to be put on the committee and work it like a politician on election day.

Review your consortium agreements. Those sometimes archaic dusty documents entered into years ago can be lifesavers. If your library is a health sciences library that has entered a legal agreement with many smaller libraries to provide interlibrary loans or other services, and the downsizing will somehow affect these agreements, this may be a powerful argument in your favor. CEOs never like to be blindsided at statewide hospital association meetings during which their colleagues confront them regarding service cutbacks. The question comes to mind of "How will it look when we don't fulfill agreements that you signed?" It may be a good idea to run these documents past the hospital's legal council to make sure they are in order. When you need them, they should be as correct as possible.

PROTECTIVE HELMET:
THE NUMBERS OF YOUR LIFE

In your desk drawer, at all times, should be the local organizational studies that prove your library saves your hospital real money every year. You do not have such studies? Why not? At the last hospital I worked at, I did a study on producing slides in the AV (audiovisual) darkroom as opposed to farming out slide production to local vendors. Even paying salaries and supplies, there was a $20,000 savings to the organization. Then a downsizing occurred.

One of the middle managers who was part of the cutting squad got me into a room alone. She had a goal of a certain amount of people gone in her assigned area. She said, "We could always lay off the AV staff." I said, "That would mean a loss of $20,000 to the hospital the first year after the cutting. It would not save the hospital a dime. It is more cost effective to produce slides in-house than it is to farm them out to vendors. Here is the study I did to prove it." I gave her the study, and said, "Cutting the AV staff would lose money for the hospital, not make it. I'll take this to the board if I have to. It is a bad decision. I have alternatives, if you care to hear them." (Note to novice managers: If you must pin a person to the wall, give him or her an out, but only the out of your design.)

You would consider the case closed. I was asked the same question several times during the course of the downsizing as cutters got more nervous and their goals more out of reach. "Why don't we cut the AV staff?" The retort was always, "That would be fiscally irresponsible and I have the studies to prove it." The AV staff stayed.

That is just one example of a study that could save your job. How many searches do you do every year? Have they contributed to patient care? Shortened length of stay? Saved a life? Why not do a study that proves this? Elicit information from physicians. Keep track of responses. If you can prove that in one instance you changed behavior, shortened the time to a correct diagnosis, or helped get a patient an improved treatment, it could translate into a study that would prove the department's worth. With one day in the hospital costing thousands and a readmission costing tens of thousands, suddenly library services can be vital services.

When you train staff in computer use or MEDLINE use or some other issue, do you do evaluations? How do you know if your training is good or helpful? Do you follow up? You would be surprised how easy it is to get feedback by calling people who have taken your courses and learned from them. Keep a record of it. Some librarians do more training than computer services at their institutions. Can you say, for example, that you trained x number of people in search engines or MEDLINE use? If an outside consultant came in to do this training, it would cost the hospital x number of dollars. If you weren't there, would computer services need to hire another trainer? How much would his or her salary be?

Here is an interesting tactic. Has a search you have done stopped a malpractice suit from happening? Can you prove it? Can you prove you stopped just one lawsuit a year from materializing? It is hard to prove a negative. With the high cost of health care, if one physician admits you made a difference, it could translate into the cost of your department for a year or two. Have you worked with quality improvement (QI) lately? If QI takes credit for reducing the length of stay by better treatment of hip surgery patients, for example, and you did a particularly good job on the research, maybe you can take part of the credit.

If anything, librarians do not take enough credit. We work behind the scenes, but our work has great impact on our organizations. Blow your own horn. Take credit when it is due. Do you save your thank-you notes?

Is your journal collection fiscally smart? The $100,000 you spend on your 400-journal library translates into how many interlibrary loans at $12 or $25 apiece? You should have these numbers at your fingertips. How much would a document-delivery service cost the hospital? Suddenly the cost of your interlibrary loan clerk does not seem so high.

GREAVES OF STEEL: BENCHMARKS, FLOWCHARTS, ORGANIZATION CHARTS, AND EVALUATION SURVEYS

Do you benchmark? Do you set exact time periods for having vital work done? Can staff rely on you to fulfill certain promises? If you do not benchmark your vital functions, now is the time to do it. Select three or four of the most important things you do, whether it is literature searches, interlibrary loans, or some other function vital to customers. Find out what the industry standard is, if possible. Find out what your colleagues are doing. Set a higher standard for your organization. Keep records. Every six months, or every year, check to see that your work falls within the benchmarks. Make adjustments if your benchmarks are not up to standards (and make sure your customers' needs are part of that standard). Survey your customers to see if they are happy with the benchmarks after they are in place.

Why a higher standard? Simple. Later in the book we will discuss mergers. Mergers pose special problems for the librarian. When you and another librarian are on the chopping block it may be your benchmarks that save your job. Benchmarks can be considered part of those studies you conduct as part of your job.

Have you evaluated your services recently? Sent out any surveys to target groups and made changes based on their comments? Get in touch with your users. Talk to them informally and through surveys. Find out what they want and give it to them if at all possible. You want your users very happy with your services just before a downsizing. They may be the same people who decide the fate of your library.

Is your paper house in order? (Are you the master of your domain?) All your vital processes should be flowcharted to show their efficiency. You should have an up-to-date organization chart to show how all the players relate to each other and who reports to whom. Your policy and procedure manual should be up to date. All your papers should be in order. This will come in handy later when you have to make your big presentation.

MORE ARROWS TO FILL THE QUIVER:
THE LITERATURE

Hospitals are study-driven organizations. Physicians will not change their practice unless they see a study confirming that the new treatment is superior to the old one. Administrative weasels won't do anything unless they have the numbers to back up their claim. We as the information gurus of our organizations supply those numbers and those studies. We work the literature every day to prove and disprove one theory or another. Why aren't we using the literature to prove the need for us? Some studies prove that hospital libraries are vital. Next time you are fired at, fire back with the literature.

McGowan, J. "For Expert Literature Searching, Call a Librarian." *CMAJ* **165(10, 2001): 1301-1302.**

Fire that first salvo with this recent article (actually a letter) in the *Canadian Medical Association Journal*. In the letter, the president of the Canadian Health Libraries Association makes a very cogent argument for medical librarians being involved in all areas of medical research, especially after the tragic events that happened at Johns Hopkins University when someone in a clinical trial died.[12] Remember, defend yourself as well as your library. Library literature contains examples in which librarians have successfully defended their collections only to find their jobs gone.

Klein, M.S. and Ross, F.V. "Effect of Online Literature Searching on Length of Stay and Patient Care Costs." *Academic Medicine* **69(June 1994): 489-495.**

At three Detroit hospitals, librarians studied whether using MEDLINE searches had an impact on length of stay and patient care costs. They took 192 test cases in which a MEDLINE search was requested and compared those cases to 10,409 similar cases by DRG (diagnosis-related group) in which a MEDLINE search was not done. The conclusion reached was that those cases where MEDLINE searches were conducted during the first half of hospitalization statistically had significantly lower costs, charges, and lengths of stay than those whose searches were conducted later.[13] The bottom line to physicians: do MEDLINE searches early and often. (Note: This study has recently been criticized for its research methods. Use it at your own risk.)

Homan, J. M. "The Role of Medical Librarians in Reducing Medical Errors." *HealthLeaders Online.* **Available at <www. healthleaders.com/news/feature1.php?contentid=38058>.**

Librarians who address the real problems at their hospital are effective librarians. Michael Homan, who is Director of the Libraries for Mayo Clinic, makes a strong case that medical librarians can significantly reduce medical errors and reduce the 100,000 deaths in hospitals every year.[14]

Marshall, J. G. "The Impact of the Hospital Library on Clinical Decision Making: The Rochester Study." *Bulletin of the Medical Library Association* **80(April 1992): 169-178.**

Often cited, this study shows that MEDLINE searches can change medical decisions; thus, it is possible to postulate that a MEDLINE search can lower length of stay and provide better care.[15] Along with the King study, it is a strong argument for good medical library services.

King, D. N. "The Contribution of Hospital Library Information Services to Clinical Care: A Study in Eight Hospitals." *Bulletin of the Medical Library Association* **75(October 1987): 291-301.**

This study of eight hospitals in the Chicago area involved a total of 176 physicians and showed that hospital libraries do make a difference in patient care. Use this quote at your next managers' meeting. "Nearly two-thirds of the respondents asserted that they would definitely or probably handle their cases differently as a result of the information provided by the library."[16] Libraries make a difference.

Lindberg, D. A., Siegal, E. R., Rapp, B. A., Wallingford, K. T., and Wilson, S. R. "Use of MEDLINE by Physicians for Clinical Problem Solving." *JAMA* **269 (June 23-30, 1993): 3124-3129.**

Written by Dr. Donald Lindberg, the director of the National Library of Medicine, the conclusion to this study says it all. "MEDLINE searches are being carried out by and for physicians to meet a wide diversity of clinical information needs. Physicians report that in situations involving individual patients, rapid access to the biomedical literature via MEDLINE is at times critical to sound patient care and favorably influences patient outcomes."[17] Little else needs to be said. Rapid access to current literature makes a difference in medical care.

Schacher, L. F. "Current Clinical Issues: Clinical Librarianship: Its Value in Medical Care." *Annals of Internal Medicine* **134(April 17, 2001): 717.**

The clinical librarianship program you started many years ago may one day save your job. Schacher details the history of clinical librarianship and, more important, the studies that show our value to clinical care.[18] Stop at this study for the ammunition you need to fight the battle.

Palmer, R. A. "The Hospital Library Is Crucial to Quality Healthcare." *Hospital Topics* **69(Summer 1991): 20-25.**

Palmer (then executive director of the Medical Library Association) eloquently states the case for the hospital library in the electronic era. Palmer showed that hospital libraries are cost effective and directly impact patient care in a positive manner.[19] It is always good to cite studies outside your own library literature, such as this one in a publication read by the board at many hospitals.

Hammond, Patricia and Priddy, Margy. "Hospital Libraries Are an Economically Sound Investment." *MLA News* **341(November/December 2001): 1.**

The title says it all. Hospital libraries are good financial investments for a number of interesting reasons. Hospitals get a lot of "bang for the buck" with a good hospital library run by information professionals. Not only do libraries improve patient outcomes, but an argument can be made that they are no-cost continuing education for staff, they decrease the cost of research projects, they are an effective low-cost recruitment and retention method (prospective top-notch medical staff expect their employers to provide top-notch research services), they decrease the line item for books and journals by putting them all in one place, and they are low-cost public relations and community health programs.[20]

Baldwin, Jerry. "Mn/DOT Library Accomplishments." *Transport Connect.* **Available at <http://www. transportconnect.net/top.html>.**

Did you know that a special library could provide an estimated 8.4 million dollars in reduced costs and added value? This is an added value for benefits-to-cost ratio of 12:1.

Although not a hospital study, this is an eye-opener because it is a detailed cost-benefit analysis that would be difficult to refute.[21] If a transportation library can save its professionals millions of dollars a year, how much could a hospital library save the hospital? Is a trained librarian searching for information more cost efficient than a physician or nurse? This study shows that a trained librarian is a good investment. The next time you have to do an end-of-year report, consider using this format for a report that will knock their socks off.

This is by no means a complete list. Any article written by Gertrude Lamb or Ralph Arcari on the value of clinical librarianship is a good place to start and forms a historical basis for the articles stated here. Many more articles out there prove that medical libraries play vital roles in hospitals. You should review the literature on a regular basis and use these studies to prove your worth. Sometimes in our rush to use the literature for others in the organization, we forget to use it for ourselves. If librarians don't value the literature, can we expect others to value it?

COUNTERING THOSE SLINGS AND ARROWS

You have heard the refrain before and it is sure to come up during a downsizing. Someone will say, "Why do we need a library? All the information we need is on the Internet for free." You may not realize that it is an old argument. In the 1980s, I tried to get a referendum passed in a town in New England for an addition to the local public library. During the meeting, one selectman turned to another and said, "Why do we need a library? I own a book." I turned to a colleague who was also listening and said, "I know for a fact that he has never opened it."

The "Why do we need a library when all the information we need is free on the Net?" argument is many times the first attack of the budget cutters and should be countered quickly before it becomes part of the mob's chant. This argument may be countered in two ways. It is implied that librarians are not needed because "It is all on the Internet." Studies have shown that American companies spend $107 billion a year paying their employees to search for free stuff on the Internet.[22] In other words, "free stuff" costs American corporations $107 billion a year. The average knowledge worker spends as much as eight hours per week looking for information. Cruising the Net could be costing your company millions. Consider the saying that goes, "I spent four hours saving ten minutes by trying to find something on the Web."

In health care, librarians have worked long and hard to make medical databases such as MEDLINE user friendly. But, does it make sense or is it cost effective to have a physician search MEDLINE? Wouldn't his time be better spent treating patients? Should the highest paid personnel in your institution be searching or should librarians who are trained to search be searching? Even if you do not consider yourself a great literature searcher, shouldn't you be the one training staff to search thus saving the hospital thousands, perhaps millions, of dollars a year in wasted staff time doing bad searches? If your information systems department is the authority on equipment, shouldn't you be the authority on medical knowledge resources? Is it too far-fetched to state that just as most hospitals now have a chief information officer (CIO), most hospitals should have a chief knowledge officer (CKO)? Is this the model for the new millennium as opposed to the informationist model proposed by the *Annals of Internal Medicine*?

Of course, anyone can search the Web now using Google or AltaVista. And anyone can do brain surgery, right? I feel we have gone too far in trivializing what we do (searching) to the detriment of our own profession and our users' needs.

The second point of a bad argument is that "It is all on the Internet." A study was done recently that showed that 62 percent of business leaders believed that the business information they needed was available on the Internet. In reality, only 28 percent of the leading twenty publications that major companies refer to most often were on the Net; 82 percent of the sources studied do not provide free, publicly accessible archives of articles. Studies prove that paying professionals to search the Web for high-quality, targeted information is far more cost effective than relying on the amateur searcher.[23] Any information professional who learned to search in the 1980s can attest to the high price of failure. Back in the days of Dialog and BRS, a failed search could cost the hospital hundreds of dollars. Instead of dollars, today think of the problem as time and one can see it bleeding out of an organization as staff do poor time-consuming searches.

In other words, it is not on the Web, and if it is, you need a librarian to find it. In the remake of *Shaft*, the hero asks a villain, "Do you think that makes me less dangerous or more dangerous?" (referring to Shaft being without a badge). So, too, we can say to our critics, "Now that the Internet has expanded information exponentially, is it less or more important to have a knowledge expert to make sense of it all? Can you say physicians should be making decisions without the best possible information? Is that good for malpractice?"

FINAL DEFENSE: MILITARY INTELLIGENCE

I had a director who said to his managers, "If you hear anything about the board, pass it on to me. If they order a pizza at Bella Roma, I want to know about it." That director knew the benefit of good intelligence-gathering. He was able to anticipate small problems and deal with them before they became big problems. He also never forgot a board member's birthday or the age and names of their children.

Although it is difficult to know everything in an organization, it is advisable to know enough and understand the subtle and gross forces at work in your organization. In one organization, an LTA's (library technical assistant) job was to take money to the finance office. His other job was to come back with information, as the finance office is a hotbed for rumors in the organization. The cafeteria can be an excellent source of information. If you do not eat there, casually mention to your staff that any interesting information that they hear would be appreciated. Good intelligence means reading the hospital board minutes religiously and anticipating the board's needs. If someone at a board meeting brings up an issue, send that person a packet of information on that issue with a note saying you heard he or she needed some information. Get the board in the habit of using you just as you got the physicians and nurses into the habit. They are your stakeholders.

By the way, it is never a bad idea to cozy up to board members, especially the ones who are techies and love to talk about books, computers, or information science. You could help them with their information needs and at the same time educate them to the importance of the library in the hospital. Never use them to end-run your boss. It would be better to tell your boss what you are doing, reassuring him or her that you are doing both your boss and your department a good turn.

NOT-SO-DIRTY TRICKS

You need excellent information flowing in, but you also need excellent information flowing out. You are your own information ministry. You dispense information about the library every day to staff, patrons, and administration. This is all part of that positive attitude that was touched upon earlier. You do it without thinking. You see someone in the hall and he or she asks how things are. Do you say, "Great. We just acquired a new database that will help marketing contact potential customers for the hospital." Or do you say, "It's Monday. Wish it was Friday." Do you say to your staff, "Those jerks upstairs are cutting my budget again." Or do you say, "Here are the facts as I know them. We will work through this because you are a great staff. You have always done great things and I expect nothing less."

Educate your boss early in the process. Get on the committee that interviews to hire new chiefs of departments and vice presidents. This accomplishes several purposes. It makes you an insider. You have firsthand knowledge of new people coming on board and can screen out people who may not be library friendly. If you interview a person, you can casually mention how wonderful the library is and give examples (plus your business card for follow-up questions). When the new person is hired, he or she will not know many people in the new organization except that intelligent, friendly, helpful library director he or she met during the interview. You have an "in" with all new management. This can be an incredible advantage because you may be able to get your agenda to him or her before anyone else does. The new hire may be grateful to you for helping him or her get the new position. The new hire sees you are a mover and a shaker in the organization if you are on the interview committee. You are blessed many times by this tactic.

Every time you perform a great search or get a compliment for helping someone do you say, "Thank you. Would you do me a favor? Could you write a note to my boss telling him how much I helped you? I would really appreciate it." Consider your boss's file on you to be an interactive file that you can build with positive statements that you make sure are there, or the negative statements from other people when there are complaints. No matter how good you and your staff are, there will be complaints.

A young friend in junior management with a Fortune 500 corporation explained it all to me once: "When you do something good, it's an 'atta boy.' They slap you on the back and say 'atta boy.' You need a lot of 'atta boys' because eventually there will be an 'oh shit.' That is when something goes really wrong. You need at least five 'atta boys' to counter one 'oh shit.'" How many "atta boys" do you have handy?

Ever notice your successful colleagues? The successful ones manage the news about themselves and their departments. You hear only about the successes, never the failures. It is a very good habit to get into. Manage your own news. Always positively advertise yourself in your organization.

It can be a simple tactic, and it doesn't have to be a dishonest one. A positive spin does not need to be an immoral act. Always advertise your successes (and your library's) in the company newsletter, company e-mail, and the like. If you don't have anything else to say at a meeting, tell the group about the article you just got published. Advertise yourself as a winner. Promote yourself. I find that libraries are very personal things. Your personality may be the telling factor in whether your library succeeds or fails. Think of yourself as a winner. You will find people will consider you a winner. Finally, does every piece of paper that you generate have your organization's name on it? We do the searches, get the interlibrary loans, produce the slides, bibliographies, and a host of other things. Who gets the credit for these good works? Do they appear in conference rooms and doctor's offices and nurses' stations by magic or does someone's hard work enter the equation?

Recently, I took over a graphics department. I asked the staff, "Why isn't the department's name on the materials you create so well? You do great work. You guys are unsung heroes of this hospital. Why doesn't anyone know this? Why don't you advertise your services?" Their response was extremely interesting. They said, "The former director wouldn't let us claim credit for our work by putting our name on our stuff. We weren't allowed to advertise our services. He said we all belong to the same university, so we don't deserve credit."

It was no coincidence that the department was languishing with little work coming in. That former director missed an important point. Even in a university in which everyone is on the same team, different members of the team need stroking. They need to have pride in their work. They need to have people demand their talents. If stroking is the only compensation, then stroking must be provided for morale. Where is the incentive in any system in which no merit raises are given for exemplary work and seniority is far more important than the quality of your work or taking pride in what you do? These people were being underutilized. If you have pride in your work, you take credit for it and make sure people know where it comes from. This not only generates more work but gets the credit where credit is due.

Now that you are armed, you are ready for the first assault, the announcement. Your resolve will be tested here in ways you never imagined. If you survive, the fun is just beginning.

Beatings will continue until morale improves.

Seen on a pirate-themed T-shirt
in Ocean City, New Jersey

Chapter 3

Hostilities Begin:
The Announcement

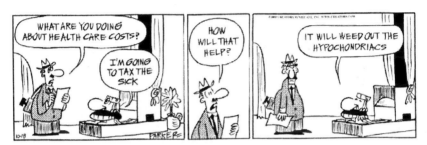

Barzini will move against you first. He'll set up a meeting with someone that you absolutely trust—guaranteeing your safety. And at that meeting, you'll be assassinated. Now listen—whoever comes to you with this Barzini meeting—he's the traitor. Don't forget that.

> Don Corleone to his son Michael
> *(The Godfather, Part I)*

Michael Corleone could tell you that those big meetings with competing managers are never fun. Someone you trust comes to you and proposes a meeting. It is important to note the order of events. Barzini moved against Michael Corleone first. Even in the Mafia it is important to move first before your opponent gets the chance. Ever go to a meeting and swear that you are the only one who was not divulged the outcome beforehand? That it has all been decided before you enter the room? I have gotten several odious jobs that way. You find you have been betrayed. In the end, it comes down to your friends versus theirs. Someone is fast on the draw and someone is slow. In the background, someone starts playing Italian opera music. Someone gets shot. Sometimes many people get shot as many old scores are settled at once. There is always much blood and gore. People die in fanciful posed ways with ballet grace. After a while, the smart actors learn to avoid parts with Italian opera music if they want to be around for the final credits. Like Michael Corleone, we all want to be around for the final credits with some of our ideals unshattered.

THE PARANOID ZONE

Certain things will happen just before a downsizing or other BCE. At first, you will brush off the rumblings as corporate paranoia, but the signs are still there. Anyone familiar with this process will tell you a healthy case of paranoia is not a bad thing at certain times. Look for the following in your organization.

- *Major decisions are put on hold.*[1] These decisions could be anything from a computer system to a new staff member or hiring a replacement for a staff member who has left. You notice a dead zone—a sudden slowdown. This is one of the many predictable dead zones in the process. For the manager, it is an early warning sign. Suddenly all processes slow down or grind to a halt. Upper management knows what's going on, but you are out of the loop.
- *You find you have much less influence than before.* Before, you could get what you need just by making your case for it. Now, you are put off or stalled. Upper management may be in numerous meetings or suddenly off-site for days at a time. Your calls to your boss go unanswered. The rumor mill is working overtime. Public affairs may not put out much public relations at this time or may put out stilted, very positive announcements. It is decidedly like the forest before a violent storm when all of a sudden the birds stop singing and the bugs stop buzzing.
- *You are not kept up to date on new developments.*[2] Managers are definitely out of the loop during this period. Your travel budget may be cut without warning. Education is not a priority at this time. Upper management may take those funds to use for the consultants. You just won't know it at the time. Someone from manage-

ment may ask you for a list of your employees' job descriptions or duties. They may ask if the library is being utilized. (As if you will turn around and say, "Nobody comes in here anymore. I wish you would just close the place down.") Suddenly they are very interested in how many hours you are open. They will ask you if you have utilization figures. Now is not the time to wish you had done a utilization study. In a pinch, you can pull some figures from your online databases either by yourself or have your vendor do a quick sort and computation. If you don't have the figures they need, say "I will have them on your desk tomorrow." These questions are like the scouts feeling out your defenses before the big battle.

- *When you get feedback, it is mostly negative.*[3] Upper management likes to keep employees off their game before a downsizing. You won't receive a lot of praise for your accomplishments right before a downsizing. It is hard for upper management to explain praising you one minute and laying you off the next. If you miss an objective, you are dumped on as never before. It could be a small goal for your department or a major initiative, but if you miss it you hear about it. Once again, administration is looking for excuses. Be very careful during this time. Make all your goals. Try to handle a problem with a patron locally and quietly.

HOW IT WILL HAPPEN

This is how it will happen: All the managers will be told (not asked) to be in the auditorium at a certain time. Mandatory meetings are never good. Or, you will be required to attend an off-site meeting. Usually these meetings are held publicly so upper management can state its case. Usually the presentation is well scripted, which is very important to upper management. The survival of the corporation may be at stake. Administration tries to make sure that everything goes smoothly.

Rumors may be rampant in the organization. This is a bad sign. If upper management cannot keep a lid on its communications, it is an early sign of trouble. It may mean that some administrators are not "on board" the plan and are complaining to their staff about it. Your own staff may be buzzing like a honeybee on a new flower. This is one of the things that dooms a downsizing. Some members of the administrative team are just paying lip service to the plan. Beware of saboteurs. If anyone makes negative comments about the plan to you, remain noncommittal. Upper management is very testy at this time. They don't need distractions from seditious staff. This is not the time to play rebel. If you hang with the wrong crowd at work (and you know who they are), stay away from them. Do not make yourself an easy target.

If you run the AV department, whenever an important meeting is planned, have your staff find out what is going on and report back to you when they set up the LCDs and audio for the meeting. If any handouts are lying around before the meeting, they can be perused beforehand.

An important rule of downsizings is: If they ask you to stop by the auditorium at a certain time in the afternoon, it is a small downsizing. If they have you meet at a conference center away from the hospital for a day or two, it is a big nasty downsizing. Expect blood to flow in the streets.

The reason for this is very simple. It is a matter of economics. Basically a direct ratio exists between the money set aside for the downsizing process and the amount they want to cut. Funding a downsizing takes a great deal of money. The board must approve a certain amount of funds for consultants, workbooks, overtime for overtime and replacement staff (people must still be taken care of while you, the administrative staff, physicians, and all the nurse managers are in a room somewhere for days at a time), etc. You can't stop a hospital for a few days to restructure. Sometimes the paperwork alone takes weeks of nonstop work to complete. Consultants don't come cheap. A downsizing may cost the hospital a half to a million dollars.

If they are willing to spend a half million to cut positions, disrupt the workflow of the entire hospital, and have valuable staff bail during the process (staff resignations are a fact of life at this time as staff become disenchanted with the process), how much return are they expecting for their half million? $10 million? $20 million? If they have set aside enough money to fund a day at a conference center, a catered lunch for 200 with salad bar and dessert tray, and have paid for high-priced consultants, they are looking to cut a significant part of their operating budget. Guess who is a part of that operating budget—a nonrevenue-generating part? Kind of makes you feel like you are going to the buffet, but are actually the main course.

WHEN IT WILL HAPPEN

An interesting point to consider is when to expect a BCE. One study showed that 55 percent of all mass corporate downsizings happen on Tuesdays. Why Tuesday? It is conjectured that most corporations like to hand down the bad news on Mondays when everyone is fresh from the weekend, but they can't seem to get the paperwork in on time. Is this humor or a real comment on the efficiency of most American corporations? Actually, no one knows for sure why so many layoffs occur on one day of the week. You may want to make a mental note: don't attend meetings on Tuesday.[4]

Interviewing for a new job? Waiting for a call from a corporation? Another point of interest is that Thursday is the hiring day. Most corporations like to call prospective employees on a Thursday to offer them a position so the chosen candidate doesn't have the weekend to decide. In a tight labor market a competitor might make an offer in the meantime and steal the candidate away.[5] Some corporations are very predictable. Others are more predictable.

WHAT TO LOOK FOR
AT THE ANNOUNCEMENT

How do the administrators present the information? Are they nervous? Nothing dooms the process like a nervous, unsure administration. Staff can smell fear. Is the presentation clear? Concise? Do you understand the process? Are the handouts clear? Is the paperwork doable in the time frame allowed? Are the goals achievable? If upper management cannot articulate what they need to keep the company viable, how can staff be expected to carry out their requests? What does it show about their planning process if the numbers are unrealistic?

Will a support team be in place to assist you with any questions you have? Where are they getting their data? Is their data honest? Should you check their numbers? (Might be a good idea, but don't challenge them in public.) You are the information professional here. Analyze their data just as you would analyze a case study or meta-analysis. Who are the consultants? Have they done a hospital downsizing before? Hospitals are unique businesses so be very afraid of any group that comes into the hospital without experience in health care.

If the consultants do not offer the information, the first question you should ask is, "What other hospitals our size have you consulted at recently?" Be very afraid of an administration of B-school thugs who would hire them if they do not have similar experiences. Would you hire a surgeon who never did that particular delicate surgery before? E-mail the librarians at the hospital where they worked and get an honest opinion about how the downsizing went. Many librarians do this before the JCAHO surveyors come calling. It can be useful to do before downsizings, too. Your battle-hardened peers are great sources of information. Prepare a written list of questions so you don't forget to ask something vital. Quiz them on any effective buzz-words that the consultants like to use so you can use these in your plan (hot buttons). Ask them for any successful plans they drew up. If you do get any plans (they are usually confidential), notice the style and organization. Call and get more than one opinion. Someone may have had positive experiences with a consultant team. Someone else may have had very negative experiences. Try to sift through the emotions to get to the information beneath. You may accidentally push some hot buttons during your interview. Be ready for anger and a host of other strong emotions. Note: offer your services to the consultants. They may need your information-gathering skills to help answer staff questions.

Critiquing the announcement is very important. Don't let shock or surprise disconnect that great brain and those analytical skills that have gotten you where you are. "Shock and awe" was a favorite business tactic used by consultant weasels a long time before it was ever used on the battlefield. You need to understand this and not be a victim of it.

Know what's going on so you can adequately deal with it. Ask yourself some important questions. Who are the players here? Who is doing the announcing and what is their stake in the process? Are there people up on the dais who are not part of the management team? Why? What talents or skills do they lend to the process? Are you friends with people on the dais? How can I benefit from helping those people? How can I be helpful and supportive to administration during this process?

Ever notice that no one tells a manager he or she is doing a good job? (As a manager, you are familiar with this. How many times have staff come up to you and said, "Thanks for getting us that new water cooler.") Maybe your niche at this time could be upper-management support. You may want to look at the downsizing literature and send upper management some good articles. In this manner, you might be able to motivate and manipulate the downsizing discussion in your favor by sending the articles to a friendly administrator. You may want to take a more active role and volunteer for any committees that management deems necessary. This is not the time to be an outsider. Get inside as far as possible. The people who make the ultimate decisions seldom cut themselves. Upper management may make token cuts at their level but usually save the knives for middle management and line workers. Question: How many cleaning staff employees do you have to fire to equal the salary of one administrative lizard?

CONSULTANTS

Chances are, at the announcement, you will meet the consultants for the first time. Consider them the sons and daughters of Satan and act accordingly. If your typical MBA got his or her degree by going through a soul-sucking machine that sucked most of the humanity out of him or her, then the typical consultant gleefully volunteered to go through the machine a second time to make sure every shred of humanity was gone. They make automatons look lifelike. Their sole goal is a financial target. They are seldom around for the aftermath.

You may consider this harsh, but consultants are not in favor at the moment. One of the great business writers of all time, Machiavelli, knew all about consultants. In his classic work, *The Prince,* he warns civil authorities against waging war using mercenaries. This advice is especially useful today. Machiavelli thought that since they were doing an odious job just for the money, their motives were suspect and their true agendas hidden as were their loyalties. Machiavelli recognized only two kinds of mercenaries (consultants): the skilled ones would win you the war but never leave and would try to attain more power, and the unskilled ones would lose you the battle. It is interesting that in his scenario, either way you are out of power in the end.[6]

Today, mercenaries (consultants) don't fight battles for city-states. They recommend downsizing and outsourcing. These two activities are not self-limiting for the consultant. It is like buying cocaine from a dealer who will advise you to do it only once. After a downsizing, there may be less business activity because the new staff can't handle their new responsibilities or the wrong people were let go. Thus, more downsizings are needed to stop the bleeding. The consultants have started a vicious circle that only they benefit from.

When dealing with consultants remember:

- As Machiavelli said, "A prince who is not himself wise cannot be wisely advised." No matter how great the consultants, upper management got the hospital into this mess and they must accept the advice and make changes.[7]
- They are not your friends. Consultants have financial targets to meet but you are just that, a financial target. They will leave you with a mess to clean up. Be professional with them if they need assistance with literature searches. Provide them with the information they need but be warned that the support of your career is not in their mission.
- Beware the good cop/bad cop ploy. For reference, see any episode of *Law and Order.* If one consultant seems to be your dear friend and one seems to hate your guts, watch out. They may be trying to manipulate you into doing something you will regret later.
- Watch out for mission creeps. They are supposed to help you cut 10 percent and suddenly they are suggesting 15 percent. They may be trying to make up for a failure to cut in another department by overcutting in yours.[8]
- Make sure you get the first string. Consultants like to do the bait and switch. They host the kickoff meeting with their senior staff and suddenly you are dealing with someone right out of B-school with no hospital or library experience. If their eyes glaze when you try to explain to them the necessity of ILL (interlibrary loan) procedures, ask for another team. You are not there to train the greenhorns.
- Be wary if consultants try to get more consultants on board. They sometimes lowball their quotes to management to get the contract, then try to get more of their colleagues on the project at hospital expense.[9]

If the consultants don't teach you new stuff, give you expertise that you didn't have before, something is wrong. Their job is to give you new knowledge so you can do your job better. When consultants give you practical answers instead of pushing a hidden agenda, a downsizing can work.

HOW TO TELL YOUR STAFF:
COMMUNICATION 101

If you don't communicate with your staff, you are in big trouble. Who processes the interlibrary loans or catalogs the books? Who would know what kind of processes could be eliminated or streamlined? Your staff is vital at this time. And, it is a two-way street. You are vital to your staff, too. They may be very scared and upset. They will need conversation and reassurance from you. It is time you enrolled in Communication 101.

If you asked most managers to rate their communication skills, most would say they do a good to excellent job communicating with their staff. Their staff would disagree. Just as people learn differently, so do people hear, process information, and understand differently. A single missive delivered in the same way may only reach a small part of your staff. You may be actually sowing misinformation in your organization by your communication style. That old adage about starting a rumor and listening to the end result and comparing it to the original rumor is very true. Distortion is common. Sometimes it is so common that the original rumor and the final rumor have little in common. The more people who get the news, the more it is distorted in the telling.

Many managers know the drill. They are promoted from the line because of their skills in their jobs. In other words, they are technologically proficient at their job (and love doing what they do). In the library trade, this may mean you are a great reference librarian or technological services librarian. Now you are promoted to management. You are expected to have totally different skills as if by magic. Instead of doing the job, you manage the people who do the job (and you may be very envious of the people who are doing the things you used to love to do). New managers are expected to be managers without much training. Have you learned to communicate with those people you manage?

Don't worry. The consequences of not communicating with your staff are only poor cooperation and coordination, lower productivity, tension, gossip, rumors, and increased turnover and absenteeism. Maintaining excellent service during a BCE is very important. Your department must be perceived as efficient and necessary. The manager you supply a journal article to today may be on the team that is in charge of cutting staff in your area tomorrow. Your staff must be focused enough to get the job done during these turbulent times.

The following are a few suggestions for improving communication with your staff:

- Realize that communication is a two-way street. Don't just talk. Listen.[10]
- Put more emphasis on face-to-face communication.[11] Follow up those paper missives with a little walking around (of all the management styles I have been taught, management by walking around has been the most useful). Staff like to see their boss. Ask staff if they understood what you sent them or if you can clarify something.

If you have staff who are assigned certain areas or head certain departments, have them start looking at cuts in their area as soon as possible. Make them report back to you with their findings. If staff have a say in the cuts and have buy in, they are more willing to go along and be supportive.

Some ideas for improving communication include:

- Concentrate on creating credibility with your staff. Managers who do not build credibility aren't trusted. Anything you say will be dismissed as untrue or management hype.
- Get publications out to staff regularly. Don't just rely on that once-a-year emergency publication but send out information on a regular basis. Consider a monthly staff newsletter.
- Take selected staff to subsequent meetings. Sometimes they will hear or pick up things you will miss. Trusted staff can be invaluable in helping other staff understand what is going on. Don't just rely on yourself. After the meeting, talk to the people who went to the meeting with you to make sure you are all on the

same page. A big problem with taking people with you is giving out conflicting information to staff who were not there. Remember you are the boss. If you make staff responsible, expect them to be responsible.

- Give staff every piece of paper you get from upper management that you can. This helps establish credibility. If you are not holding anything back, it is more likely you will be trusted.
- Hold daily staff meetings if it helps. Don't assume your staff know what is going on. Communication is vital at this time. You need to combat the rumor mill. Some vicious rumors may be floating around. Once again, listen to your staff when they tell you rumors and if you can't refute them with facts, go to management and ask for clarification. It is common to hear, "We are all going be fired tomorrow. I just heard it from housekeeping." Your staff need to know you are working hard for them. There can't be enough good information. Studies have shown that if you communicate with staff effectively, they will have a sense of control during the process. If they have a sense of control, they are less likely to suffer from survivor syndrome after the downsizing is over. Once again, an ounce of prevention at this early stage is worth a pound of cure later.

THE LIBRARY STAFF AS TRIBE

A tribe is defined as an aggregate of people united by ties of descent from a common ancestor, community of customs and traditions, and adherence to the same leaders. Consider your library staff as a tribe. You spend more waking hours with these people than you do with your own family. You bicker with them. You have your friends and, regrettably, your problem children. When attacked from outside, it is amazing how quickly the tribe pulls together. You go to their important events such as weddings and baby showers. They are invited to yours. If a death occurs in the tribe, the entire tribe mourns.

Ever notice that most true tribes have an oral tradition? Very little of the how-to-do things are written down and one or perhaps two people keep the traditions of the tribe. (When was the last time you updated your procedure manual? The thing about accelerated change is that by the time you update the manual, the procedure has changed again.) The tribal storytellers have fantastic memories for what happened to the tribe in 1986 and why a policy was instituted. This tribal historian can be vital at helping you put this BCE in context of past BCEs. If you are relatively new to the organization, the tribal historian can help you understand why situations are the way they are before you change them to the way they should be.

Now may be the time to adopt some of the attributes of the more successful members of famous tribes. Ever watch the television show *Survivor*? Some would dismiss it as just another piece of pseudo-reality television trash. I find it a fascinating study in group interaction and imagine hundreds of sociologists are taking notes while the contestants are voting each other off the island.

Look at the successful contestants. They run the gamut from old to young, black to white, and female to male. They do have some common traits worth noting to anyone going through a downsizing (besides the ability to tolerate starvation). They are providers. They go out and get stuff for the tribe. The final contestants are usually the food gatherers, cooks, or other quiet, capable, hardworking individuals. What do you bring to your tribe that is of value? Does the tribe know it? They are friendly and bond well with people but are not aggressive, bossy, or obnoxious. They know when to be quiet and let other gamers make the mistakes. When people are loud or obnoxious, they do not confront them. They play the game. They are careful in how they make alliances but when they do, they are honorable within the confines of the game. They are aware of possible threats and deal with them when they need to. Regrettably, backstabbing is a part of the game.

Game playing is a big part of downsizing. Don't be voted off the island. Support your staff during this early announcement time. They will be frightened as any tribe would be when confronted by something new. They will need a lot of support and reassurance. Fire up the old compliment machine at every opportunity. Even if you don't feel particularly upbeat, be upbeat around staff. Donuts and other comfort foods are always good for staff morale. That side trip to Dunkin' Donuts on the way to work may turn out to be a lifesaver.

Studies show that certain staff will need more counseling than others. People in different jobs respond to the news of downsizings differently. Part-time staff are many times less connected to the organization due to their off-hours status. This group has been shown to be the most nervous about job cuts and feels under the ax during the entire process. Make it a point to stay late and talk to these staff members. Reassure them that they are considered as important and necessary as any other staff member. Challenge them to come up with ideas to improve the library and cut costs. Make sure they get the same information and have the same ability to ask questions as the full-time staff.

The attitude of your staff is very important. If your staff as a whole feel that they have some control over the situation, they will cope better (control coping) than staff who feel the process is out of their control. If staff feel they have no control, they will practice escape coping. They will start to cause problems at work. The quality of their work may suffer. They may not come to work on time. They are the first to bail out and look for other positions, thus causing you major hiring and retraining problems. It is extremely difficult to replace anyone who leaves during a downsizing.

It is important to create control in their lives and relinquish some of your authority over the process. This can be quite difficult if you haven't trained staff to think independently. The size of your hospital can be an important factor in staff stress and insecurity. Staff at large hospitals feel more vulnerable than staff at small hospitals. The big cuts occur at the large hospitals because the numbers look so much larger.

Length of employee service to the hospital is another factor to keep in mind. Staff with seniority feel they have little to worry about. Staff who have just been hired feel at risk of being the first laid off. Tailor your presentations to reassure these staff members.

You have a very difficult job as leader of the tribe. You are middle management. You support your own tribe, but your loyalty is to the greater tribe—the corporation that pays your salary. As such, there are things you must do and things you should never do. You should always be supportive of your hospital/corporation. If you say negative things to staff, they will take your lead and be negative. It is almost wish fulfillment. Don't say it; you may get what you wish for. Even small cynical statements can backfire. It does not help anything to voice negative statements in front of staff.

Along with this, you should never say anything negative about upper management. You are upper management's line leadership. As such, it is your job to carry out their policies. This is your job. It is why you are paid. It is extremely counterproductive to criticize upper management in front of staff. How hard will your staff work to effect successful change in your organization if you are negative about the process? If you can't support their decisions and don't believe that those decisions are good ones, it may be time for you to dust off that résumé. Don't make a bad situation worse by your attitude. If you have questions or concerns about the process, express them to the upper-management team.

Some clever bargaining goes on during this early time period. One library manager was called into the administrator's office to talk about the announcement. They talked in general terms about what the library director could do to trim costs and meet targets. When the paperwork finally came down to the manager, he was shocked to find that his targets were based on the "off-the-record" cuts already being made and the administrator taking the credit for the cuts. Remember you are firmly in the grip of the weasel zone. Things will happen in that gray area of management as people cut corners to make their quotas. They are under a lot of pressure at this time. People under pressure make mistakes.

An extremely important thing to remember is never give anything away early. If an administrator asks, "Where do you think you can cut/lay off?" Your response should be, "I'll have to look closely at the budget and how any cuts would effect certifications and accreditations, and get back to you after the paperwork comes down. I need to look at my mission and how cuts will effect the mission." You must stay in control of your part of the process and not let others control you. To borrow a phrase from *Survivor,* "You have to play the game and not let the game play you."

Six important points must be remembered during this period and during the announcement period in general:

1. Never discuss specifics before you have to.
2. Never give up anything ahead of time.
3. Never give up too much (you get no extra credit).
4. Never give up too little (if the target is 3 percent give 3 percent). Cutting less will get you in a world of hurt.
5. Think about what allies you can draw on. Now is the time to think about what groups you have synergy with and how this

may help you. Be creative. Could nursing education or human resources be useful allies?

6. Don't make any promises yet. That will come later.

Feeling better about the whole downsizing process? You have all your facts and figures in place. Your résumé is up to date and your mission statement is clear and righteous. You know every certification and accreditation that pertains to the library and have your studies in place to fight off any frontal attacks. The benchmarks show you run a world-class organization. You have successfully negotiated the shoals of the announcement and are just waiting for the paperwork from the consultants and the first planning meeting of managers to start. Now breathe a sigh of relief.

You have calmed down a nervous staff by effective communication and assured them that the library will function smoothly while you are in nonstop meetings for days on end by delegating many of your day-to-day duties, realizing that this is the most important step you as a manager will ever take. You have informed your most frequent and demanding customers that you will not be available for a while and told your staff that they must bear the work burden while you fight the good fight for them. You have surveyed the downsizing literature from libraries and business before you begin. You are now ready to sit down and really create a better organization based on the principles outlined in this book. You are looking forward to turning this potential disaster into an opportunity to make changes you have always wanted to make—to sweep out the old. You can envision a twenty-first-century virtual library.

You sail forth from your office right into a thick pea-soup fog of nothingness. Your ship is caught in a dead calm with no wind to fill your sails. You can't see the stars to navigate your course. Your food stores are rapidly running drastically low (running low on chocolate bars). Your staff is planning to mutiny (guess who gets to walk the plank?). You have just entered the Phony War Zone. The best is yet to come.

What do I know? I am only a librarian.

Jet Li, *The Black Mask*

Chapter 4

Phony War Syndrome (PWS)

> All war is deception.
>
> Sun Tzu

And so it begins. You stumble in complete shock to your office after the announcement is over. Several colleagues greet you along the way and you don't really see or hear them. You mumble greetings. Numbers and scenarios swim through your head. You consider how many support staff you will need to lay off. How much of the journal budget to slash. You think to yourself, "Well at least the rumors are over. We now know what we are dealing with. The worst is over." Wrong! Welcome to Phony War syndrome.

This is a chapter about nothing. It is the hospital library equivalent of a *Seinfeld* episode. What can be said about nothing? As Jerry Seinfeld proved, a great deal can be said. Seinfeld milked nothing for many, many seasons of television humor. Can you just hear him doing stand-up saying to the crowd, "And that dead period right after the downsizing announcement. What is that all about?" Regrettably, there is no laugh track during the Phony War. It is a time when many battles are won and lost through inaction or false moves. You are fighting your enemy in a deadly haze, swinging your sword at phantoms.

PHONY WAR EXPLAINED

The term *phony war* comes from a time in World War II, roughly October 1939 through April 1940. The Germans had invaded and taken Poland. The British Expeditionary Force landed in France but no immediate fighting began. The French waited at their "impenetrable" Maginot Line. Each side tried to end the war through negotiation, but Germany would not relinquish Poland and negotiations fizzled. For more than six long months, two great armies stood poised staring at each other but few shots were fired. Everyone just waited.

Many opportunities were lost during this period. The French did not fortify their Maginot Line.[1] The army went to ground, thinking their position impregnable, not understanding the implications of a mobile mechanized army at their borders. They prepared to fight the last war instead of preparing for the next one.

Isn't that just like some managers? They prepare for new incidents based on their own experiences, not realizing this is a totally new occurrence. The sitzkrieg of the French (German slang for the phony war period) was totally unprepared for the blitzkrieg.

In the past few years, many companies have downsized. To the uninitiated, it would seem like a straightforward process. Upper management sets a target for reducing overhead by cutting staff or operating expenses. The announcement is made. After a planning period in which the details are worked out, middle management makes the cuts. People are laid off. The survivors take over the duties of the people who are gone. After a company mourning period, life goes on, productivity goes back up.

Would it surprise you to know that the time between the announcement and the actual downsizing can be as long as a year to two years? That six months of nothing happening is not a long time in weasel-ese (the language of corporate consultants)?

What does that mean to you and your staff? Emotionally, everyone's life is put on hold for a year or longer. Should you buy that new washing machine? You might be laid off. Go on a vacation? You might need the money if there is a downsizing. Fix up the house? Might be laid off and have to move. (After the downsizing is over, you suddenly realize that you have 1,000 chores to do that you couldn't find five minutes for before.) Can you afford to send your children to that private college or will they have to go to a state school? Just don't know. Nearly every normal thing you do is put on hold. It can emotionally rip a family apart. People crack under the strain. Many turn to the Employee Assistance Program (EAP) and seek counseling. Some turn to very unhealthy outlets such as drinking and drugs. Managers try to protect their turf and are not afraid to point the finger at others. A lot of "take him not me" happens. Plans are made so that favorite staff are protected, thus taking the objectivity out of the process. This period brings out the worst in many.

Expect absenteeism to be high during this time. One study showed that sick leave was twice as high during a downsizing.[2] This you will need to plan for. If this is especially irksome to you, bear it. Staff need to deal with the stress. You are not the only one under pressure here. It is not a bad idea to suggest counseling to staff who seem especially troubled.

At work, it is no better. Start that new project? Why bother when there is a downsizing? Finish that project you started? Not if you are going to be fired anyway. A librarian in the field said that he thought with budget cuts there are also definite issues about starting new projects when you don't have the funding yet or when your funding is threatened. Should you start a project if you might not be able to finish it?

Your telephone calls to other managers are not returned. There seems to be reluctance on their part to solve any problem or assist you in any way. Physicians and nurses stop asking for literature searches. No research is done. Everything grinds to a sudden halt.

If you thought that the atmosphere was spooky right before the announcement, it is downright *Nightmare on Elm Street/Halloween/ Friday the 13th* afterward. The halls of the hospital are surprisingly vacant. No laughter comes from offices at this time. There is no chatting between offices. All the joy has been sucked out of the organization. Work is not a place many want to be. People snap at each other. Staff don't want to be caught in the halls not working. Administration is far too busy to worry about team building.

The natural tendency is to hunker down. People dig foxholes and stay in their offices. They talk to colleagues on the telephone in hushed tones. Some staff show incredibly immature behavior. One library director said recently that he had one staff member who was worried about the downsizing. She came into his office every five or ten minutes all day long to tell him something. After she came in to tell him she was moving journals on a shelf behind circulation to a lower shelf, he screamed, "Carol, you have to stop this. Your job is not in jeopardy." Until he said something, she did not realize that in her nervousness she was running around the library like the proverbial chicken.

Staff meet in the cafeteria and in hushed tones play the downsizing game. The downsizing game involves guessing which employees will lose their heads when the ax falls. Everyone plays this game. No one is excluded. This game involves more aspiration than anything else. It is the "wouldn't it be great if (insert name) was downsized" game. Sometimes the real villains in an organization would be revealed if upper management would just listen to a few staff rumors. Staff's wish list may be very different than management's list. Make no mistake, management has a list. Many old scores get settled during this time. Employees who have embarrassed themselves or not met quotas are prime targets. In the completely fair, manager-driven process that is corporate downsizing, the goats always lose (unless protected by management).

OPPORTUNITIES

Consider the French at the start of World War II. Instead of fortifying the Maginot Line, they just waited, hoping the Germans would accept a negotiated settlement. In other words, they prepared for the best and ignored the worst. In war or business, this can be disastrous. They missed a valuable opportunity to prepare for war. How many men could they have trained to fight and get to the front in six months? Are you missing a valuable opportunity to profit from the stasis? What benefit can stasis be? Consider if everyone does nothing and you do something great.

When General Oliver Smith found that his army was trapped behind enemy lines during the Korean War, he was accused of retreating. His comment will live forever in the history of military annals. He said, "Retreat, hell. We're just advancing in another direction." It is time to pick a new direction and advance. Four case studies supplied by hospital professionals come to mind.

CASE HISTORIES

Case History No. 1

In 1993, a colleague of mine was in the middle of a downsizing dead zone when he decided to use the time wisely. No requests for literature searches were coming across his desk. No research projects. In a matter of days, his work had dried up like a small stream in the desert.

So with a lot of time on his hands he sat down at his computer and taught himself html programming. It was not that hard to take an html code, break it up, and insert new pictures. His hospital did not have a home page, as the Web and the Net were in very early development. As a good manager should, he recognized that the Web would be a great mode of marketing the hospital and getting consumer health information to potential customers/consumers. He recognized a paradigm shift before anyone else in the hospital. Computer services did not have a single staff member proficient in html. Marketing and public affairs didn't have any plans for using the Web. They did not see the paradigm shift to Web marketing until it was too late.

The librarian wrote a very basic but well-designed Web page for the hospital. It was the second or third hospital Web page in the state at the time. He was far ahead of larger hospitals in the state. Of course, the page prominently featured the library. He found a local Freenet to host the page. After it was tested, he asked for ten minutes of the CEO's time and wheeled a computer into his office (after getting approval from the librarian's direct supervisor). It was bold move time. The CEO's eyes lit up like a Christmas tree when he saw the Web page. In a matter of a few days, the librarian was featured at several board presentations demonstrating the Web page for board members. For three years, he administrated the Web page for the entire hospital. Vice presidents and chiefs of service had to come to him to have information loaded. It significantly increased the library's value in the organization. The library was seen as being proactive and future-directed. His reputation as a visionary was ingrained into the mythos of the organization. Whenever there were planning committees formed to make technological changes, his name was first proposed. The librarian in question took initiative and used the dead zone to take the high ground. Any military strategist will tell you that the most important thing you can do in warfare is to have the best position and make the enemy come to you.

Case History No. 2

Another library manager looked around during the phony war period at his hospital and saw that a manager was just fired in a department that had a lot of synergy with his own (an AV department). He made a proposal to upper management to take that department under the library's umbrella, thus saving the hospital the cost of a manager. The librarian worked hard turning around a demoralized group of people and championed their cause whenever possible. Every success that the new department had was blasted in the company publications. By the end of the phony war period, the library manager could show that he had done a very creditable job turning around an unproductive group of employees, giving them direction and purpose. He fared well during the downsizing. He wrote off the former manager's salary as part of his downsizing effort even though it occurred before the downsizing. He was seen as a valuable effective manager who saved the hospital money and managed one of the best-run departments in the hospital.

Case History No. 3

An Australian librarian in a personal communication said it so well it can't be improved upon. She said, "I have learnt that to be still is to be abolished. So although services slow down, we are busy finding details of the new agency (to replace the one that is reorganized). There is usually a change of minister too. So that means keeping the top brass informed of the curriculum vitae of the proposed minister. Because we are seen as keeping (them) up to date, there is recognition of our role in the new set up. Within a few days (of the reorganization), I am making contact with the 'new brooms' to find out their information needs and it goes on from there." That is a librarian who will be keeping her head while others around her lose theirs.

Case History No. 4

A librarian reported that her slowdown was a time when the corridor to the library was closed to install new floor covering. The library had to be closed for four days. Instead of sitting around on her hands, she planned an outreach activity and took the library to the people. She e-mailed all the community health centers and services connected to her hospital and arranged for a road show. She made up library information resources folders and went out and visited, demonstrating databases, distributing information packets and explaining library services. All the sites have networked computers, so the librarian was able to register new users right at the sites. After the carpet was replaced and the library reopened, she saw a 91 percent increase in people from the off-site facilities using her library. Her road show was so successful that it has become an annual event.

Consider, when a downsizing or slowdown occurs at the main hospital, maybe the off-site facilities could use your services. Set up a minilibrary at an off-site location and keep your momentum going.

OPPORTUNITIES FROM OTHER LIBRARIANS

When quizzed, other librarians suggested writing articles, doing research, or taking online classes/courses to improve your position. One enterprising librarian suggested that a downtime is a good time to remodel the library Web page. This would be a good project as Web pages seem to grow old very quickly and a beautiful, very functional one would look good to administration at this time and remind them of your worth. That librarian added a Spanish-language section for consumers, a disaster preparation and response area for professionals and laypeople, plus a section for nursing and medical students.

Some librarians suggested training for whatever will come after the downsizing is over. It is still early in the process, but this is very good advice. When others are floundering in the aftermath, you may be poised to get off to a running start if you have a clear view of what is to come. Researching a grant may be a good idea. If you are very lucky and bring some money into the organization during a downsizing, you will look very good (and that money may offset some of your required cuts). Remember it takes a year for a downsizing to roll out. You can apply for many grants in a year's time.

One librarian reminded me that downtimes are always followed by manic due-yesterday days. What can you do to prepare for the manic times to come, even if it is photocopying more literature request forms to be ready for the deluge? If literature searches dry up, maybe you could proactively search the literature, pull great useful articles, and have them ready to hand out when the downsizing is over.

Technical services librarians have suggested many ways to keep busy during downsizings, such as verifying access to the electronic serials. (A new job that never goes away. Publishers seem to change passwords and access points at an alarming rate.) Catch up on claiming missing issues. Work is always needed on bibliographic records. Even in the electronic age, a cataloger's work is never done.

THE BUSINESS MODEL

We are not the only profession to deal with slowdown during downsizings. From the business literature these suggestions have been gleaned:

- Don't blame your customers when things slow down. They are dealing with the same stresses you are.[3] It is tempting to get angry when colleagues don't bother to stop by or use your services. Consider that you will need to work with these people after the dust settles.

- Stay in touch with your customers. Send out e-mail notes asking them if they need your help or follow up with research already done.[4]
- If a shift in business focus is imminent in your organization, plan for that new focus by doing preliminary research in that area.

THE INNER CIRCLE AND POSITIONING

We can assume that if you were caught off guard by the downsizing announcement that you are not a first-level player. You need to penetrate the inner circle quickly. You need to become a first-level player or align yourself with the first-level players. How do you become one of those architects of the culture, values, policies, and practices of the organization?

The following five simple keys are suggested for reaching the inner circle.

1. *Be the best in your profession, excellent at your craft.* We have discussed ways for you to be effective in your job. Attaining mastery of your job shows you are ready for greater responsibilities.[5]
2. *Keep your ego in check.* If you are in a position of authority in your hospital, if you have the CEO's ear, don't abuse this privilege. Don't brag to colleagues or whisper little secrets.[6]
3. *Stop thinking tactically. Think strategically.* Think about your organization as a whole, not just your part. See connections, see possibilities, and envision outcomes outside your area of expertise. Trusted advisors are more than smart. They are wise, competent, and creative.[7]
4. *Tell it like it is. Don't be a "yes" person.* Good advisors tell the truth and have the courage to express it.
5. *Do the right thing.* Although unethical practices are mentioned in this book, your integrity is extremely important. Who would trust a person who is unethical?[8]

If the inner circle at your organization is rife with politics, ego, backstabbing, and grab-the-gold ring mentality, you may want to stay away. But if it is a place where you can do yourself, your library, and your hospital some good, go for it.

You also need to create "good buzz" about yourself in a hurry. Think of yourself and your library as a product that you want everyone in the organization to want. How do you create good buzz? In the business and finance world, they know to create demand; you attract attention and engage the prospective client.

There is a one-minute positioning method that is used to get a sales message before prospective users that can be very effective. You know your clients (do your market research), know what they want or need, and start a dialog that engages them. Instead of introducing yourself as the person who does searches, try starting with the words, "You know how . . ." You could say, "You know how you generate a lot of questions in your practice but don't have time to answer them before the next patient comes through the door? I'm the person who will supply you with the information you need when you need it." You could also say, "You know how malpractice rates are going through the roof? We supply you with the information to practice state-of-the-art medicine." How about saying, "You know how doctors spend many years in school and training and then have limited time in which to maximize their earnings . . ." The power of this type of dialogue in terms of sales psychology is that it focuses on the prospect, not on you. It is far more important that you are interested than that you be interesting. It also emphasizes the prospective client's problems. One business source says, "Remember, prospects don't care how much you know until they know how much you care."[9]

Now that you have engaged your client, you can say, "What I do is . . ." "What I do is help doctors make the best decisions so they practice the best medicine." This second reply answers the most important question in the prospective patron's mind, "What's in it for me?"[10] Before health care professionals trust you with their information queries, they want to know how you and your services will make them feel better, happier, more confident, and secure. Now that you know how to position yourself before a single client, consider ways to position yourself before the entire organization.

You may not be able to write your hospital's first Web page or consume a department, but when no one else in your organization is shining (while hunkering down afraid, paralyzed by fear and uncertainty), you will shine all the brighter if you do something great during this period. You must be calculatingly bold during the phony war period to set yourself up for what is to come. You must be in the best possible position before you plan and implement your changes. Think of positioning as authority. You need authority and the reputation as a superstar.

It must be perceived in the organization that you are among the best and brightest, a shining star far too valuable to lay off. A success will give you that position—that valuable high ground. For further information on high-ground thinking, read *The Killer Angels* by Michael Shaara. This fictional account of the Battle of Gettysburg is one of the finest war books ever written. It is also an excellent textbook of business management if one reads between the lines.

When going into a merger with another health care organization that has a librarian, some librarians would throw in the towel thinking that the director of the larger library will always win. This may not always be true. One librarian may sit on his or her laurels while the other librarian is jockeying in the organization to be seen in the best possible light. Do you do a lot with limited funding? Can you prove your staff is more efficient? Do you have great relations with your medical staff? Are your benchmarks better than the other person's benchmarks? Can his or her studies match your studies? Are your surveys and evaluations better than the other person's surveys? Can you prove your customers like your services more? Now you begin to see why benchmarks and surveys are so very important. Are you more in tune with your hospital's needs? Do you have unique talents such as training staff or writing articles for publication that someone else does not have?

A caveat should be mentioned here. Be very careful when "attacking in a different direction." Select a project, have a plan, and stick to it. Make sure what you do has a real benefit to the institution. Some people think their manic activity will be mistaken for achievement and run around like ADHD (attention deficit hyperactivity disorder) children off their medication. They don't make decisions. They just make noise and pay the price of looking unprofessional or erratic at a time when negative scrutiny is the last thing they need. Nothing succeeds like success, but a failure at this time can be fatal.

Now is a good time to read "out of the box" to prepare for the innovation to come. If you read just in your area of expertise, you will think like everyone else in that area. What is a management book anyway? Could a Martha Stewart book give you insights into human nature? Would Rudy Giuliani's best seller *Leadership,* which details how he dealt with the crisis of 9/11, be a great management book for times of crisis? Could a child-care book that assists you with dealing with immature staff behavior be considered a management book? A technical article in a videogame magazine may lead to a new idea for a wireless information system. (Want to learn about the new technology? Borrow *Electronic Gaming Monthly [EGM]* from your teenage son or daughter. This publication explains complex technology issues in clear language that even an adult can understand. Their clear explanation of the basics of wireless Internet connectivity was excellent.) Read *PC Magazine* to find out what consumer technology is coming down the pike.

I have already recommended *The Killer Angels* by Michael Shaara, and *Dilbert and the Way of the Weasel* by Scott Adams to understand the lowly motivations behind many people's business decisions. His book is chock-full of e-mails from corporate drones who have observed amazingly bizarre corporate behavior. It seems that the *Dilbert* cartoons are no more insane than the actual corporations they satirize.

Another wonderful management book that most librarians might overlook is Joe Torre's *Ground Rules for Winners: 12 Keys to Managing Team Players, Tough Bosses, Setbacks, and Success.* Anyone who can hop into the stress-filled cauldron of major league baseball and succeed with one of the worst micromanaging, question-your-every-decision bosses in the history of the universe, a hostile media constantly nipping at his heels, homicidal fans demanding his blood, a tradition of success to live up to (the gods of the port looking down from Valhalla), and a multinational staff of neurotic prima donna players should be read cover-to-cover and studied closely. The chapter on dealing with difficult bosses should be mandatory reading at every business school in the world.

While we are on the topic of overlooked great books, if you ever plan to write a book, read Conrad and Schulz's *Snoopy's Guide to the Writing Life* to understand the joys and frustrations of writing for publication from a literary beagle's perspective (and that of some fine contemporary authors). Who can deny that, "It was a dark and stormy night" is one of the great opening lines in all of literature? I can sympathize with Snoopy on the whole issue of rejection notices.

Now is the time to do what you are paid to do—to think like a manager. Be innovative. Analyze your systems, recognize the new paradigms, and change what needs to be changed. Take the best of what has been done in the profession and use it creatively. Plan. Take chances. How well do you plan? Implement change? Get staff on board?

On the other side of the equation, how well do you lay off staff? You shouldn't ignore this nasty little task of the manager during a downsizing. How well do you train staff in their new duties? You are about to plan as if your livelihood depended on it. It does.

Chapter 5

Planning Your Campaign

Never underestimate the power of stupid people in large groups.

a) Louis XVI
b) a downsized employee
c) demotivator library

The secret of managing is to keep the guys who hate you away from the guys who are undecided.

Casey Stengel

Planning is never easy. If you are not good at gazing into crystal balls or conjuring up the ghost of Melville Dewey, you need good information on what the hospital library of the future is going to be like. You will not have the option of re-creating what you already have. Although not set in stone, the following are some trends in hospital libraries that you should be aware of.

Sit down and read out of your field a bit (as recommended in Chapter 4). It could be anything from management, business, a news weekly, or investment magazine, but you can't think out of the box without different knowledge. Clearing your head is important. You are about to imagine the future. Close your eyes and try to see what the future of hospital libraries will be, based on the trends you have recognized in the literature.

What we will be doing in this chapter is creating a business plan based on your actions in Chapter 2. (Why do you think you created all that nice paper of a mission statement and did all those studies?) You need a strong argument when you go into that presentation meeting. Your business plan will give you that. By using the arguments that the financial "wonks" use, you will defeat them at their own game.

TRENDS IN LIBRARIES

This could be a difficult section to write. Anything said could be out of date in a matter of weeks, thus dating the book. If I say that personal digital assistants (PDAs) are the wave of the future in special libraries and this vision does not happen, then I seem like a fool. If I don't say anything useful, you will not find the information you need to plan, and the book will find itself on the remainder rack all too soon (the literary equivalent of a movie so bad it goes directly to video). So what do we strive toward in trying to keep our organizations in the know? Are you investing in copper wire when high-bandwidth wireless technologies are right around the corner? Have you bought databases on CDs only to watch the information go on the Internet?

An important trend to consider when you reinvent your library is the education needs of your organization and how you can support those needs. At the turn of the twentieth century, the public library was the "university of the masses," helping to educate and Americanize the flood of immigrants that arrived on our shores. Back then, the library did what no one else was doing by preparing these people to be part of the American workforce.

Today, libraries are confronted with a similar mission. Change happens so quickly that it is extremely difficult for staff to keep up. It is postulated that instead of ten or twenty years between major technology breakthroughs, change can happen in many fields in as short as three years—a mouse's life span. There is no time to go to a class for a few months to learn a new skill or keep a certification. Staff must learn on the go. Some staff are going back to education after a long layoff. Staff members who come into the library and ask where the card catalog is will need a lot of training. With online classes, distance learning, CEs (continuing education) on the Net, etc., your new role may be the education center of the hospital. Consider partnering with nursing education or medical education or any other education departments in your hospital. This is the time to become proactive, to understand that the mission of the library has always been to dispense information and educate users whether the information is wedded in the world of Gutenberg or Gates. We must also remember to choose technologies that are in our customers' comfort zones, not necessarily in ours. We must remember to market ourselves as mediators of the technology and not just the technology itself.

Consider what you offer and how it differs from what your customers can get sitting in their pajamas at home surfing the Net. Do you offer AltaVista, Google, and Yahoo!? Can you prove you offer something that they can't get anywhere else, even if it is just superior training?

Consider the virtual library as the proverbial horns of a dilemma. On the one hand, you work hard to make information access seamless to the user. They can hop on the Internet, get what they want (using your Web page as their portal), link to full text, and print off the article at their desktop. Have your library and your visibility suffered because you have engineered your value out of existence?

Consider the full-text revolution. Ten years ago, the average patron was delighted to get an abstract with a citation list. Now, they expect full text. Will content analysis be next? I receive more and more requests for "the answer." Professionals have less and less time to review reams of literature. They need people who can review the literature and take the next step by deciding what is relevant and what is not, what will work and what will not in a clinical situation. Will the informationist touted in the *Annals of Internal Medicine* be the next big leap in hospital librarianship?[1] Will you be able to make the jump or do you lack the necessary skills to review reviews and test tests?

The following are some five-year information format trends from the OCLC (Online Computer Library Center):

- Over the next five years, librarians will continue to be faced with managing an incredible array of content in a rapidly changing array of formats. This is a major point. The information revolution is an incredibly messy thing (a neat revolution would be an oxymoron on the order of jumbo shrimp). In many hospital libraries, 35 mm videotape journals exist next to paperbound journals next to online journals. Have the old technologies gone away? Have CDs completely replaced cassettes? Have DVDs replaced videotape? One of the major problems of the new century for hospital information professionals will be the storage of information in many different formats.[2]
- Many library patrons are quickly adopting the new information retrieval formats, such as PDAs, cell phones, e-books, tablet PCs, etc. For the librarian, keeping up with these changing formats will be an increasingly difficult task. A surgical resident told me that he wanted it all on his PDA. He wanted it now. He didn't want to have

to walk to radiology to view an X-ray or go to the lab for test results. It should happen when he wanted it and where he wanted it. If this is your customer, you will be hard pressed to meet his demands.

- Tools, services, and technologies that did not exist ten years ago are shaping expectations of access to information. When you are planning, factor in big bucks for development and replacement, even though you may not have any idea what the new technology will be. Be assured, there will be new technology and your patrons will demand it.[3]

- These new patron demands must be balanced against tighter budgets and smaller workforces. Doing more with less will be the mantra for the future. Patrons expect full text, but administration never understands that electronic databases cost money. Educating upper management to these issues will be a never-ending, full-time job.

Looking at trending in the scholarly materials area, the *Survey of Academic Libraries 2002* edition found that book purchasing by academic libraries was down 8 percent from the preceding year. University press hardcover sales fell 26.8 percent in August 2002. Library purchases of university press books were down 12 percent during the same time period.[4] In the journal area, several seers predicted that research journals would be published almost entirely online. In 1994, there were fewer than seventy-five peer-reviewed electronic journals. By 2002, 75 percent of the journals in *Science Citation Index* were online. In a recent survey, 84 percent of the faculty and students at Drexel University stated that they preferred e-journals to print.

The scholarly article is migrating away from traditional print to e-journal. Soon, the very idea of an issue will have started to sound ancient. If there are no issues, will there be journal check-in as it is known now? What will that mean to the journal and binding staff?[5]

Another interesting trend is the rise of e-print archives. E-print archives are repositories for electronic versions of papers (self-archived by the authors) that are made available to the scholarly community prior to publication. ArXiv, the physics e-print archive at Cornell University, is estimated to increase from its present 210,000 preprints to more than 385,000 a year by 2007. There are presently more than 15 million downloads of arXiv content each year. Could this trend signal the death rattle of the scholarly journal as ballooning journal prices ensure yearly cutbacks and send librarians searching for alternatives?

According to Dissertation Abstracts International, a strong trend is emerging toward electronic production and away from creating new paper dissertations. The number of new paper dissertations is expected to decline over the next few years, while a British Library study predicts that by 2007 at least 50 percent of all theses will be submitted electronically.

More than five billion pages of copyright-cleared articles are currently available for use on the Web. This figure will double by 2007. In other words, if you are in an academic library and don't have an active e-reserve program, you are very far behind the curve. According to a U.S. Campus Computing Project survey, as many as 56 percent of U.S. college courses could be available via course management systems (such as WebCT and Webcasting) by 2007.[6]

Now that you have a clear idea of what the future will hold (if it is clear to you, you may have a future in the stock market or betting on horse races; at least you will be recognized as a visionary in the library field and be swamped with offers to speak at conferences), you can turn that clear view into a vision that your staff and your customers will embrace. Vision motivates your planning process because you have to know where you're going before you find a road map.

VISION STATEMENT

From your mission statement, your study of the future of technology and libraries in particular, you should by now have an idea of a vision for your library. Your vision differs from your mission. Your mission statement tells people why your organization exists and how you will accomplish this task. A vision statement should be clearly focused on your customer with your staff as the prime mover.[7]

Your vision statement also leads you into the future. It sketches a picture of the library's desired future in a few paragraphs. Where are you taking your organization? If staff and customers know the direction the library is going in, all will be happier. Can you answer the question, "What will be different in the hospital in three to five years in terms of information dissemination because our library exists?" If nothing will be different, lock the doors now. Another question you must answer is, "What role will our organization play in creating that difference?" If you do not envision a vital role, once again lock the doors now and save yourself some grief. This stuff is not for the faint of heart.

The great thing about a good vision statement is that it gives staff a picture of what they can accomplish. In nonprofit organizations, there is little incentive built into the system. Staff do the same job every day with little change in their day-to-day routines. If library management is not good at communicating the goals of the library, staff can be disaffected and distant. With a good vision statement, staff are compelled to stretch and do extraordinary things. They feel good about themselves.

Remember the following points when crafting a vision statement.

- *Make your vision statement compelling.* Emotion, not logic, moves people to do great things. Also, successful vision statements are visual. If you write a visual image of the future, your staff will be able to connect on a subconscious level and make it their own.
- *Eliminate rhetoric.* This seems to contradict the above statement but really it just calls for the right kind of writing. Get to the heart of your message. Write a sentence that every employee needs to hear, understand, and believe.
- *Don't state the obvious.* The obvious (we will check out books) is not compelling. A vision statement that says, "In the next five years, we will adapt wireless technology to disseminate information throughout the corporate campuses" is compelling.[8]

An effective vision statement ties into other people's motivations. It gets buy-in from both staff and your customers. If you do not have a clear vision of the future or if conflicting visions exist, maybe more than one vision is necessary. Don't let uncertainties hamper you. The military is famous for having a plan for every contingency. If Canada invades the United States, we have a plan in place. Libraries should adopt this philosophy more often.

SWOT-ING YOUR ORGANIZATION

Chances are your library could use a good SWOT-ing. In this case, the SWOT stands for a method of strategic planning that analyzes *S*trengths, *W*eaknesses, *O*pportunities, and *T*hreats. It's a four-part approach to analyzing a library's overall strategy or the strategy of its departments. To implement your vision, you need a good SWOT analysis. The goal is to identify all the major factors affecting your competitiveness.[9] It used to be that a hospital library was not in competition with any other department. That was before IT (information technology) came into existence or patient and nursing education came to the forefront. Even training and development may be nipping at your heels. In some ways, you find yourself in a hostile environment. SWOT helps you with that.

To help you do a SWOT analysis, ask yourself the following questions:

Strengths

- What does your library do well? Be honest; do you have a unique program? Maybe it is something that your core customers love. If you don't have a well-loved program or service, ask yourself why not. What brings your customers in by the hundreds? What should you be doing?
- How strong is your library compared to other hospital libraries in the area? Are you the smallest and weakest or strongest and most robust? One library went from weak to strong in its community by cutting back less than its neighbors. After a few years of holding the line, suddenly the library in question was a major player.
- Does your library have a clear strategic direction (vision statement)?
- Does your library have a positive work environment and what do you do to produce one? If you have a tradition of celebrating staff's birthdays or a great library issues discussion group, this may be an important strength.

Weaknesses

- What are your liabilities? Is your staff not capable of dealing with new technology? Do they fear change? Do they not work well independently? Are your night staff disaffected? The downsizing will create enormous staff problems. Don't ignore them when doing your analysis.

- What could improve your library? Be honest here. If your library is poorly lit and people cannot read the labels on books because of the darkness, write it down. Is your carpet so rotten as to be dangerous? Is the library noisy or poorly placed in the hospital?

- What does your library do poorly? If necessary, have a person who has never visited the library come in and try to use the facility. (This is referred to as a secret shopper in business terms.) Find out what that person did and didn't like. Sometimes after we have been in a library for a few years, we become so comfortable we cannot see what the consumer sees.

- What should be avoided? Is there a service that is provided by another group in the hospital that you could supply but would be duplicating? You may want to ask yourself what value you add to your organization by your unique services. If you are doing something that IT is doing and you have less time than before (with the cutbacks), you need to rethink this process.

- Have you budgeted for needed technology? If wireless is coming down the pike and you have not budgeted for the expenditure, thus weakening your library's position, this may be a serious weakness. Many librarians don't budget for future expansion. It is much easier to get a proposal passed if it has been on the table and discussed for a few years than if you suddenly spring the issue on an administrator with an "everyone else has it" argument. Don't crisis manage.

- Are you getting the funding overall to fulfill your vision? Is the library being starved by poor funding?

Opportunities

- What favorable circumstances are you facing? In the middle of your downsizing, there may be opportunities to use staff in new ways. Introduce new innovations in your library and discard the old. You have the rare opportunity to make things better by reviewing all the processes and discarding ones that don't work or are no longer needed.

- What are the interesting trends? I have outlined many interesting trends in the special library field. Pick one that excites you.
- Is your hospital entering new markets and how will this impact your library? Many times new residency programs are planned and initiated without the library having any input into the resources needed to support the residency. When the residency receives the inevitable site inspection, the library has to be ready.
- Is your library and/or hospital advanced in technology? If your hospital is one of the first in the state to have a truly advanced electronic medical record, what will this mean to information dissemination at your hospital? What will this one thing change for you? Will library services migrate to point of care information dissemination? What are your plans?

Threats

- Honestly, what obstacles do you face both internally and externally? A vice president of finance that doesn't believe in the need for a library? An aggressive department head who would love to consume your department? A lack of funding that is strangling the library? A SWOT analysis forces you to be honest about the state of your library and the hospital.
- What is your competition doing (inside the hospital, in the area, or nationally)?
- Is changing technology threatening your position? (Can you say "paradigm"?)
- Will state or federal laws impact what you do?[10]
- Consider all the internal factors. These include the corporate structure, culture, and resources.

Consider the shareholders, your customers, and competitors. External factors to consider are the political climate, technological breakthroughs, societal changes, and economic realities. Now you have a solid analysis of your organization just in time to change it. You have numbers you need to meet. Nothing makes the reality of a downsizing clearer than the numbers.

BUDGETING IN A NEW MILLENNIUM

Your budget is the numerical reflection of your mission and vision. In other words, you spend your funds to fulfill your goals and objectives. One should always reflect the other. A good strong narrative justification and your list of goals and objectives for the preceding year and upcoming year should be included with your budget submission to show how the money was spent and will be spent in a logical progression.

You have been given a target budget number lower than your present budget. Here is where the pedal hits the metal. You have two major areas to reduce expenses, your materials budget and your staff. Do you know what journals are presently being used in your library? If you cut the *New Zealand Left-Handed Surgeon Journal,* that one surgeon will make your life a living hell; but does he actually read the journal? Does anyone? A trick I learned a long time ago was how to do a "quick and dirty" survey of what journals are used in the library in any given month. Instruct the staff to put colored dots on any journals found on the tables and by the copiers for a given period of time. After a month or so, you will have a pretty good idea of what journals are being used. When that surgeon comes to you demanding that you resubscribe to that obscure journal, show him or her the lack of dots. It may not be scientific but it can be very useful.

Don't just look at the physical services. Are your electronic services draining you dry? They are becoming bigger and bigger parts of our budget but few librarians do cost-benefit analyses on their usefulness. Have you looked at usage patterns lately? Most database providers will give you usage patterns for their services to your library. If those sexy electronic full-text resources are not being used, maybe you should look at them with an eye to cutting back or replacing them with other e-journals that would actually be used. Many times libraries buy the newest high-tech solution when the paper would be more than adequate. Don't spend $5,000 for a software package when a $50 paper file would work just as well. If necessary, call your book vendors, journal subscription vendors, and e-journal vendors and ask for better bids. Explain about your budget cuts and that you do not have the funds you used to have. Demand bids from three different vendors for the same services and go with the lowest. Check to see if you are getting the best discounts through your consortia.

Are your hours cost effective? If you are open nights and weekends and no one comes in then, maybe those hours should be cut. Some would consider it heresy to cut hours. No good manager likes this, but it sometimes becomes necessary. Your wonderful suite of online services may make a visit to the library at night or on the weekend unnecessary.

When you start cutting, cut a little more than needed. If $10,000 has to be cut, cut $12,000 but only give upper administration $10,000 (with their permission). This gives you a bit of wiggle room for later when you realize you accidentally cut that favored journal or service. You will seem like a true administrator making bold decisions to give the best service to your customers. And you know what? It will be true.

A good budget not only makes sure that the money your library is given is spent appropriately, it is also a way of explaining to management that information costs real money. It can be one of the most effective reporting mechanisms you have. Administration understands numbers. Spreadsheets seem to work far more effectively than narratives to busy execs who have little time to read. That is one reason it is important that your budget accurately reflects what your library spends. Do not make the mistake of putting all your materials under one lump sum. If you do, you will not know how much is spent on books, journals, or electronic services. If those numbers are broken out, you have a more accurate reflection of how the money is spent. You will hear the refrain, "You have lots of money in the book budget; just cut it 10 percent." Little do they know that the book budget also contains the journals for the entire hospital and the online services vital to the modern hospital library.

You should not ignore the revenue side of the equation. Most administrators don't realize that libraries make money. You may charge outside users copying fees or interlibrary loan fees. The library may do a booming business from overdue books. Some hospital libraries provide services to outside organizations such as law firms or nursing homes. Grants are available for specific projects or philanthropic donations. I got a call one day from the development office at the hospital. The director of the development office said that a woman wanted to donate $25,000 to name the library after her recently deceased husband, who was a former member of the hospital board and a book collector. The director asked me if I would like to go to lunch with them and discuss the donation. I played nice. Every year thereafter, I got a check for $25,000 from her for improvements to the library and the purchase of new technology. During my tenure at the library, the woman donated over $250,000.

Revenues, grants, and donations can be a particularly thorny problem. Everyone wants to show they contribute (the library is no exception), and sometimes a good revenue source will literally fall into your lap. It is how the money is put back into the budget that becomes tricky. If it goes into the general fund of the hospital, it may be lost to the library. (Why work hard to raise money if you can't use it?) If it goes into the library budget, some financial managers would decrease the library budget by the same amount. (Again why look for donors? Why write letters to sponsors? Why take wealthy seniors to lunch?) If possible, have the development office set up a separate account and earmark the funds for special projects, remodeling, or equipment. If this is not done, the money will be used for general expenses. If necessary, work out a deal with the finance department. Some services such as interlibrary loan and copier accounts could go back to the hospital, while some monies such as grants and donations could go back to the library. Remember to have all donors write "reserved for the library" on the check.

CONSIDER YOUR OPTIONS

Have you considered all your options? You've looked at your journal costs, book budget, electronic resources, interlibrary loans costs, and staffing. Now look at your institution as a whole. When you are playing the game, use the whole board. Don't be limited to your part. Here is where good communication comes in. What are the rumors coursing through your organization and how can you profit from them? A few case histories should suffice.

Case History No. 1

A hospital library director was confronted with a difficult decision during a downsizing. He had to reduce his staff by one. There was no way around it. The particular person targeted for termination was a good, hardworking employee who was a credit to the library, although she was underutilized. She also was her sole support and needed the job. (Don't think those attributes don't enter into it. Even the coldest manager thinks about the people who work for him or her. Few enjoy firing good personnel.)

His staff told him that a staff member in another department was retiring in a few months. That person was being underutilized. There was not enough work to keep her busy. (See how important it is to have good information flowing into the library?) Assessing his staff member's qualifications with those of the retiring person and finding a match, he moved quickly and proposed to upper management that the library staff member in question be trained for the soon-to-be-open position to take over that position when the person retired. He further proposed that the positions be combined. This proposal was beneficial in several ways. The manager was able to keep the staff member part-time; thus, he did not lose or have to fire the staff member in question. The staff member was underutilized. She was a bright employee in need of a challenge. The new position would challenge her, forcing her to acquire new computer skills that would be transferable to any position she might apply for (and thus make her more employable) outside the organization. Finally, the new position was a raise in grade and gave her a substantial pay raise at a time when most people in the organization had not seen a raise in two years. The hospital library manager was seen as a proactive player with the organization's interest at heart. It was a win-win situation. Why? Because the manager saw an opportunity, quickly assessed it, and got there first. Also, he let his upper-management boss take the credit for reducing staff without letting anyone go. Note that the library manager had to be honest enough with himself to realize that his staff member was being underutilized. When he proposed the change to the staff member he was careful to make it a promotion for good work and not a do-this-or-be-fired choice. Also, he took the time to sit down with the employee and patiently explain his reasons for the changes and how the change was good for the employee.

On the downside, the librarian admitted later that he failed to discuss his plan in advance with the manager who ran the department where the job was that he was planning on consuming. The vice president who approved the plan should have checked to see that this was done, but the library manager deserves some blame for this blunder. This was politically a bad idea and could have deep-sixed his carefully laid out plan or soured the possibilities of other deals with the same manager. Part of the "art of the deal" is doing it in such a way as to not offend the other participants. The other "art of the deal" is not being afraid to make deals. What can they do? Turn you down? Are you in worse shape than when you made your proposal?

Case History No. 2

The Shining Path is a plan so audacious, so bold that it is only heard in whispers in the wind when hospital managers meet in secret. It is the sacred relic found by Indiana Jones, full of promise, magic, and dark forces. If it was insane for Lee to divide his smaller force before Hooker at the battle of Chancellorsville, attacking from the flanks and annihilating a larger force that could have crushed his own, then the Shining Path is insanity itself. It is the prayer of Jabez in action. Jabez, a man of God, prayed to the Lord one day saying, "Oh Lord, increase my territory." And the Lord did, knowing that Jabez would use the increase for the Lord's purpose.

So, too, the Shining Path shares more than a few things with each of the previous analogies. It is as dangerous as Indy's Ark of the Covenant, bold as Lee at Chancellorsville (exploiting an enemy's weakness to great advantage), and it asks for more territory like the man of God, Jabez.

It is best explained as it was performed. During a downsizing, a hospital department manager found an area of the hospital administration that was not done well. It could have been JCAHO oversight, or quality improvement initiatives, or CME (Commission on Medical Education) accreditation, but it was there and the manager found it and exploited it. She went to upper management with a plan. The plan not only called for keeping her staff but increasing it by one member. The proposal called for her to take over the task that was not being done well. She could show statistically with a strong business plan that if she handled the particular task, it would be a value-added improvement to the hospital. She could show how doing this would increase revenues significantly (or reduce expenses). To everyone's amazement, the plan was approved. (The manager was universally called a fool for proposing it.) The manager made such a convincing argument and the plan was so well thought out that upper management couldn't turn it down. It was just that good.

If General Oliver Smith was bold for "attacking in another direction," then this is General Douglas MacArthur landing behind enemy lines at Inchon and routing the North Koreans. It is brilliant insanity. I have seen this tactic work only once in four downsizings. Are you bold enough to attempt to increase while everyone else is shrinking? Can you counteract the downsizing mind-set that your colleagues are in? Do you know of a weakness you could exploit?

Could you market your library services to nursing homes in your area, thus bringing in revenues to offset your costs? Are there a lot of law firms in your area? Could you offer them a copying service for their medical information needs? Would physicians be willing to pay for an electronic table of contents service in which you set up a custom Web page with their favorite journals on it? They could peruse the page, go to their favorite journal's table of contents, and select the article they want. There are organizations such as the National Health Care Advisory Board that make huge bucks supplying upper-level information to upper management in hospitals. Are you savvy enough to cut out the middleman and supply upper management directly (thus saving the hospital a barrel of bucks)? Could your Shining Path be a proposal to eliminate outside information services and take over their duties? Are you thinking of other ways to bring in revenue or take over a job that is not well done?

This bold tactic is fraught with landmines. Knowing an organizational weakness and trying to exploit it during a downsizing may be a fast way to find yourself on the short list of downsized employees. Your cleverness may be perceived as arrogance. Pointing out flaws in upper management is not usually a career builder. Even if you survive the criticism of upper management for bringing this out in the open and get their approval to assume the task, you have to make good on your promises. Proceed at your own risk.

Now that you have a plan, you have to present it. Write the narrative, fill out the paperwork, and present your plan to upper management. How are your presentation skills? Do your palms start to sweat when you make a presentation before a large group of people? Would you rather face a firing squad than a crowd of people? Do you long for the days when librarians cataloged books in back rooms and never saw a single person all day? It is time to sharpen your skills before that big presentation. The best plan in the world will fail miserably if presented badly.

You have peeked into the future and created a vision for your library. You have SWOT-ed your organization and budgeted for greatness. You have filled out the reams of paperwork demanded by upper management. You have created flowcharts of your work processes and organizational charts of your new organization structure. You have a wonderful Excel spreadsheet of your present and future budget needs. Now you have a plan. You have to present it to upper management and get it approved before you can implement it. Some librarians are great preparers and poor presenters. Don't let a poor presentation ruin a great plan.

Chapter 6

The Big Presentation

A tale told by an idiot, full of sound and fury, signifying nothing.

William Shakespeare,
Macbeth

WRITING FOR SUCCESS

How well do you write? What is your writing style? Do you put some stuff on paper, correct the spelling errors, and hand it in? Most library school graduates are liberal arts majors and chances are you wrote a few research papers in graduate school. (When asked how I can write fiction, I explain that anyone who ever read my college term papers knows I have a talent for fiction.) Maybe you write an occasional article for a professional journal or a brochure for your library. Maybe you only write the end-of-year report and that is in the same format year after year. Before you present that vital information, you must put it down on paper in a manner that makes sense. You need a little coaching in Good Writing 101.

Most people don't realize that good writing has a theme or moral. You start with your vision or mission and go from there. In writing, this theme carries through the entire work. In other words, a single sentence should sum up what you are trying to say and all the points in your narrative should revolve around that central point. Never ramble away from your premise.

Consider our cave ancestors sitting around the communal fire. One old caveman gets up and begins to tell a tale of bravery, stupidity, or survival against all odds (kind of a prehistoric fishing story). There is a moral just like in *Aesop's Fables*. Og forgot his spear and paid the price when he took on a saber-toothed tiger. Og died. Today Og would probably be creating mission statements. Even in this age of non-linear stories there is still a story to tell. Even *The Matrix* told a story (someone will just have to explain it to me sometime). All writing is story and all writing is some attempt to tell that cultural story or history. If you remember that fact, your writing will excel, because it will have unity and meaning. Tapping into this cultural understanding is your strongest suit as a writer.

Is your writing clear? By clarity, what is meant is not just clear to you but to your staff, your boss, and someone off the street.[1] We are in a profession rich in buzzwords. Not only do we have our own library jargon, but we borrow freely from the medical and computer nomenclature, adding a seasoning of the latest business theories to concoct a tasty stew of confusing jargon. We input real time to interface with our clients' health care needs. We access online resources, downloading just-in-time data to solve a clinical paradigm. We use Internet resources to link full text to our consumers. Strip your writing of all the jargon. You are not trying to impress someone with your knowledge. You are telling a story with a moral. (If Og doesn't agree to the plan, the hospital will be liable for millions of dollars.)

Also, there is far too much composing on the computer. (Pardon the Andy Rooney moment.) Gone are the days when yellow legal tablets were used to painstakingly write and rewrite every word. The problem with the death of the legal pad is that much writing today lacks organization.[2] Sentences and ideas are diffuse and scattered all over the paper. Librarians, being natural organizers, should show this talent in the library and in their writing.

Make an outline before you write. This becomes easier to do after you do it a few times. If necessary, create a PowerPoint presentation just to make order out of your thoughts. Your thoughts will seem much more connected. Bullet points can be your paragraph headings. In the end, your writing will be much better and clearer. Don't fall in love with your prose. You are striving for meaning, not pretty words. Write and rewrite. All the great writers do.[3] If Updike or Oates are not too proud to do a rewrite, then why should you be? First, you should write, then tear apart your writing and rewrite it from a different viewpoint. Then take your work to an outside source—someone you trust or whose writing you admire, have him or her read it, and let him or her tear it apart. Don't take it personally. All writers go through this process. If it makes sense to the reviewer, it may be ready for your bosses.

Remember, your bosses are most likely not librarians, so write to them with this in mind.

Good writing is not an accident. Few great writers just put something down on paper and submit it. They recognize writing as a craft that must be worked at continually, as a pianist practices a piece of music or a wood-carver turns a block of wood into a beautiful piece of sculpture. They consciously try every time they write to write better than the time before. Revise, revise, and revise some more.[4] Your writing will keep getting better. Those reports and narratives will get easier. But don't become complacent. Keep striving to be a better writer. Try new things. Read fiction closely and try to understand what the writer is attempting to do and why. Borrow ideas from your favorite writers.

POWERFUL POWERPOINT

Most likely, somewhere there will be a PowerPoint presentation. Studies show that people learn more with their eyes than they do with their ears. One study found that 69 percent of learners prefer visual input such as charts, pictures, and animations. Another study found that visual support increased the persuasiveness of a speaker by 43 percent.[5]

If you are not PowerPoint proficient, get help. Many books have been written on PowerPoint presentations, so the basics will not be discussed in detail here. Your hospital may have a graphic or AV department and you can get help from them. First, you must remember before you create those 400 color PowerPoint slides with animation, that you are conveying a message. No amount of PowerPoint can cover a bad argument. The secret to your success cannot be found in a software package or a piece of equipment no matter how many lumens it projects. All this technology has the potential to make your life more interesting and easier, but it does not guarantee your audience will get your message, especially if the message is poorly thought out or delivered with all the grace of an Ozzy Osbourne soliloquy. Audiences are influenced by trust. As one consultant said, "People don't want more information. They are up to their eyeballs in information. They want faith—faith in you, your goals, your success, the story you tell. Faith needs a story to sustain it—a meaningful story that inspires belief in you and renews hope that your ideas, do indeed, offer what you promise."[6] The bottom line is people want to believe there is a solution. Your story should give them that solution, with sincerity and a bit of passion. Your great graphics should support your great story.

A few things to remember about PowerPoint are:

- *Color.* Color enhances a presentation. Blue is considered peaceful and clear. Green is thought to stimulate feedback and interaction. It is a restful color. Red is stimulating and a good accent color. Never use red in a financial presentation. Your audience will see red. Black is clear but can be very boring. Avoid red/green, brown/green, blue/black, and blue/purple in slides.[7]
- *Timing.* Use the ten-second rule. If it takes more than ten seconds to read a slide, then there is too much content. Try breaking the slide up into two slides.
- *Font.* Make sure your font is clear and readable. Design your presentation for the person in the last row. If it is a large room, stick to a 44-point type for headlines and 38-point type for bullet points. Check all visuals before showing for clarity and readability.[8]
- *Slide screen.* Don't clutter your slide with too much stuff.[9] You are used to viewing that slide (having created it); someone else is not.
- *Content.* Keep things short and sweet. This is a visual medium. People should not have to read a lot of text. Your job is to tell people what the story is. Use bullet points. Limit each slide to twenty to twenty-five words with a maximum of five lines.
- *Graphs.* Once again keep things simple. If you can't easily explain what you put there, break it up into several graphs. Remember that PowerPoint is supposed to enhance, not confuse.
- *Handouts.* Make handouts of your slides and distribute them before the meeting. Make sure the handouts are readable. Don't put too may slides on a page. If everything goes wrong with the equipment, you can always lecture from the handouts. It is a good idea to make your first handout color if you can. For some reason, people tend to keep color handouts and discard the black and white ones.
- *Theme.* If your theme is to sell your proposal, all your slides should support your theme.

Be warned. PowerPoint has considerable backlash. Once the big gun of presentation graphics, sales reps report that their clients are nodding off in record numbers while viewing PowerPoint. One authority said, "I'm still looking for the PowerPoint plug-in that warns us when the jaggy artwork we just imported and distorted to fit the available space is inappropriate for our audience. I'd also like to find the utility that advises me to black out my screen altogether because I've been delivering too many facts and need to close with a success story from a company just like ours."[10] They report that the old-fashioned elbow-to-elbow discussions seem to be coming back in favor as more and more clients suffer PowerPoint poisoning. If you don't have a good argument, don't expect PowerPoint to bail you out.

Before you create slides, you should:

- *Take size into account.*[11] PowerPoint is great for groups. If you are presenting to less than six people, try a more direct approach.
- *Be interactive.* Design some breaks in the action where you can ask questions and elicit responses. Test your group at various parts of your talk. Teachers use tests not just to see if you know the subject matter but also to lock it in. You have to keep your audience engaged.
- *Don't overdo special effects.* Too much eye candy can take away from your message. All the animations in the world can't cover a bad idea.
- *Have a contingency plan.* If the bulb in the LCD blows or the LCD crashes, what will you do? Do you have a backup laptop or LCD (don't try to change bulbs in the middle of a presentation). Don't let the lack of an extension cord doom your hard work.

SECRETS OF A GREAT PRESENTATION

Your presentation to upper management at a downsizing may be the most important presentation of your life. The first thing you should know about presentation skills is you should access the level at your organization. If your hospital is into sophisticated PowerPoint, don't go into the presentation with hand-drawn overheads. Understand what the group you are presenting to is looking for and do it at that level. The following are some other points to remember:

- *Know your stuff.* Practice your talk until you can rattle off the facts and figures without consulting your notes.[12] If you must use notes, just put the major bullet points on the note cards. (Remember to think in bullet points and don't try to read large chunks of boring information.) If you use PowerPoint, print off a set of note cards or handouts for yourself. Don't give your audience PowerPoint poisoning. Limit your slides to enough to get the point across. Don't underestimate the intelligence of your audience. Boring them to death will not help your cause.

- *Make your handouts readable.* It does no good to deliver an excellent presentation if your audience is busy trying to read the handouts. Also remember to include Web addresses for every Web site you refer to. It saves many questions later.

- *A week before your presentation.* Finish your presentation and present it to your staff or other group. Listen to their comments and make the final changes. If someone asks a question and you don't know the answer, find out. It may be the same question you are asked at the presentation. If necessary, videotape your presentation and critique your performance. You will be amazed by how you look on tape. You will also be amazed how many times you say "uh."

- *The day before.* Never give a presentation in a room you have not been in, using equipment you have not used before. Book the room you are speaking in a day in advance and practice your speech using the exact equipment you will be using that day. Test the lights, check the temperature controls in the room, and turn down the temperature if you can to just above freezing. Cold people stay awake. Whether a morning or afternoon program, have some caffeine drinks and light food set out for your audience before the meeting. Arrange the seating. All the physical elements should work to make your presentation the very best. Practice using the overhead or LCD projector until you can literally field strip it in your sleep, or requisition an AV tech to stand there during your presentation. Consider having a backup LCD and laptop just in case.

- *One hour before.* Set up your program. Check the lights, equipment, and all other elements and run through your entire talk at least once. By the time you give your speech, you will be so used to doing it, you will be fine. This is guaranteed to take the stress out of your talk. Nothing will be scary or foreign after you have prepared and prepared in the actual setting.

- *When you speak.* Maintain eye contact with your audience. Don't look down at your notes too often. If you do, it will seem as if you are unprepared. One famous speaker has talked about making love to his audience with his eyes. Although I suggest not going to that extreme, a smile and a sincere attitude can go far. Don't talk to your overhead projector, slide project, or laptop. Your audience is out there and that is where you should be looking. Some animation is good when you speak. Being a statue is not good. Lizards can smell fear. Too much animation is bad. Don't run around the stage pointing at things on the screen (someone may prescribe Ritalin for you). If someone asks a question and you don't know the answer, don't just say you don't know. Write the question down and get the best answer possible to that person within an acceptable time period.

- *Disarm opponents by agreeing with them whenever possible.* I once gave a speech to a group of physicians at an off-site hospital. I was warned that the physicians did not like the group I represented. There were angry people in the audience. I was told who to look for and who would be the most confrontational. I smiled at the audience. I directed my talk to the supposed opponents. I agreed with their concerns and tried to use humor to disarm the audience. They were my enemies at the beginning of the talk, and my friends by the end of it. It is a good idea to know the tenor of the crowd before you speak. If possible, quiz the speaker before you. Find out what the audience asked about. Find out what their concerns were with the speaker's plan. Compliment your audience on asking good questions; agree to all points they raise without giving up the store. Draw them out, try to understand their agenda, and try to reach a compromise.

Laser-pointer abuse should be mentioned. Some speakers can use laser pointers quite effectively. They use them to accent a point on the screen, although PowerPoint line and pointing features make them fairly redundant. Others shine them in the audiences' eyes (LASIK eye surgery, anyone?), blinding large groups of people. Some presenters move them around so quickly that it makes people nauseous. Suddenly you are on a laser roller coaster without a barf bag in sight. Some physician presenters cannot seem to keep their lasers steady.

The pointers jerk constantly in their hands. Hopefully, these physicians are not surgeons.

Another problem can be wireless mikes. If you are not used to speaking using a wireless and you need to use one for your presentation, practice with it so you are not too loud or too quiet. Remember you are wearing it. Many people forget after their speech that they are wearing a wireless and make comments after the speech that they don't want people to hear. Nothing endears you to an audience more than a comment such as, "God, I was terrible" spoken after you leave the stage.

Some other points to remember before you get up to speak:

- This is not the day to choose business casual as your clothing of choice. If those lizards wear suits, wear a suit.
- Start your presentation with a bang.[13] Just like that great action movie you have watched a hundred times or that great murder mystery novel, nothing captures your audience by the throat like a smash-bang beginning. If you ask a question at the beginning of the presentation, maybe your audience's attention will be on you until you give them the answer at the end.
- Don't change your speaking voice for the presentation. You may think that booming voice makes you sound more important. It may just make you sound phony. Your natural way of speaking will work best every time.[14]
- Always work the room.[15] Use the time before the meeting to meet and mingle with the audience and learn as much about them as you can. Include these points in your speech if you can. Also, don't run out of the room after you speak. Stay around and chat. You may have a chance to answer any questions in an informal, less-pressured atmosphere.
- Relax. Before you speak, slow your breathing down to about twelve breaths per minute. This will relax you.[16] Good speakers are relaxed. They smile at their crowd. They exude confidence.
- Use your own stories if they are appropriate. Any concept is easier to understand if you use a real-life analogy. Avoid real-life stories that ramble or don't have easy-to-understand meanings. People understand leaky pipes, car accidents, or teenager trauma. All these things make great examples. Keep the lessons short and sweet. If your story runs on for too long, their eyes will glaze over and you will lose them.

- Speak with passion. If you are not committed to your issue or cause and sound wishy-washy about it, no one else in the room with be committed either.
- Make your ending as memorable as your beginning. If you know the ebbs and flows of a narrative, you know you should finish on an up note. People who study Shakespeare know he used humor to break up the action and drama. He used it to make his drama more dramatic. A humorous pause occurred somewhere before the big action. Then he always finished his narrative with a bang. Finish with a bang.

CASE HISTORIES

Case History No. 1

Don't do what I did. (Sounds like every good lesson you have told your children, doesn't it?) Once, I had to make a career-defining presentation to a downsizing committee composed of the senior management of the hospital and some high-priced consultants. I always start my presentations with a bit of humor or a quote. For the early preliminary presentations, I used a famous quote by G. Gordon Liddy that was very appropriate. It went something like, "When asked what was the most traumatic thing about shooting a fugitive (as an FBI agent), G. Gordon Liddy would always reply, 'the paperwork.'" This is considered cute, funny, and politically incorrect.

Nervous, at the last minute I decided to use another quote. Instead of using G. Gordon Liddy, I used one from Shakespeare, *Macbeth* to be exact. I said, "This presentation is a tale told by an idiot. Full of sound and fury, signifying nothing." There was not a sound from the audience. I had just "dissed" the process, everyone in the room, and myself. Repeating the quote didn't help. Lead balloons go over better.

It took a lot of fence-mending to get credibility back after that blunder. Afterward one of the managers at the meeting said, "I couldn't believe it. We thought you insulted us with your joke. We were stunned."

Humor can be used to break the ice or emphasize a teaching point. Humor is a double-edged sword. It can cut both ways. Use the wrong joke at the wrong time, and the bomb it creates may be your career going up in smoke. With most successful humor, there is some pain or someone is made the brunt of the humor. Much humor offends someone. If you use humor in speaking before a group of people at a professional meeting, be careful.[17] Anyone who works in an academic setting knows that there is a very narrow area of acceptable humor (usually in acceptable academic humor, a white male is the brunt of the joke). Note to self: Never quote Ronald Reagan in a meeting with academics. Use a tried-and-true story or joke. Run it by your assistant or a staff member to see how it goes over. Never wing it.

Case History No. 2

One colleague explained a trick he used in presentations. He said, "You know my manager is anal retentive. He checks every number, every word for misspelling. I have never given him a presentation that he hasn't sent back to me marked in red. So I seed my document or presentation with small obvious errors. I put the wrong date on it. I misspell a word in the title. He checks all my documents, finds the obvious errors, but doesn't find where I messed up the big numbers." Don't play games. This is no time to get cute. Your presentation should be perfect. Check every word using a ruler to better focus on the line you are checking (a proofreader's trick). Check every number, then have someone else check it.

CONCLUSION

Your presentation was a success. It was well thought out and well written. Your PowerPoint presentation knocked their eyes out and your talk dazzled them. You have been given the go-ahead to implement the changes you proposed. Now you have to make your vision a reality. Implementation is where the pedal meets the metal. Can you prepare your staff for change? Decide on what to outsource and what to keep. Retrain your staff in their new roles. There is still a lot to do, so get to it. Make the tough decisions and take the heat for the dumb ones.

It is better to remain silent and be thought a fool, than to open your mouth and remove all doubt.

Groucho Marx

Chapter 7

Implementing Your Battle Plans and the Uh-Oh Factor

The nature of bad news infects the teller.

William Shakespeare,
Antony and Cleopatra

Consider this wonderful scene in the beginning of one of the *Star Trek* movies. Deanna Troi is testing for the rank of commander. She is on the holodeck doing a simulation. There is a problem in engineering (probably a core breach) and the entire ship is in danger of exploding. The only way to save the ship is to jettison the core. She will have to seal engineering, trapping men inside and thus ensuring their death. For the good of the entire ship, some crewmembers, some of them her friends, will have to die and she will have to give the order. Through the clear Plexiglas shielding, she can see her friends and knows her order will kill them. I don't remember what decisions she made on the test but she got her commander's rank. She also learned what it was like to be senior management and have to make real life-and-death decisions in which no good solution exists, just competing bad ones.

IMPLEMENTING CHANGE

Change has been jokingly referred to as what you have left after the government gets through with your paycheck. You are about to make radical changes at your library. You look around at your staff and see people burned-out by the downsizing process (looked in the mirror lately?), people near freaking out with fear over the possibility of being laid off, and people who cannot stand the thought that something is changing. In other words, they are a typical library staff. Ask yourself, "Whose responsibility is it that they are that way?"

First, communicate with them and create a sense of urgency.[1] Explain what happened to create this crisis, how it happened, and why it happened. Transmit to them how your plan evolved, what constraints you had, and what opportunities you perceive (your SWOT plan comes in handy here). It is very important that the first action you take after coming down from that heady high of getting your plan approved is to communicate to your staff. This will dispel rumors and establish your leadership. Expect to take criticism at this point. You will make decisions and you will be second-guessed. You will be very unpopular. Leadership means setting a course and staying the course. You will make mistakes but if you don't have a fail factor in your game plan, you are not planning properly.

Next, give staff time to comment and take in the change. Post the change on the staff bulletin board and ask for comments. If you don't have an open-door policy, now is the time to institute one. You must be accessible. If staff come to you, stop what you are doing, ask them to sit down, and listen to their concerns. Let them talk. If they have questions you can't answer, write the question down, and get back to them within an agreed-upon time frame.

Schedule frequent staff meetings and give your staff the opportunity to air their concerns as a group. Be prepared to be a target. Upper management is not in the room with them. The consultants are long gone. You are there to take the heat. Even if you show them where upper management made you make the cuts, they will be angry with you.

Involve staff in the execution of your plans. You may have the lonely job of coming up with the solutions, but execution of the plan doesn't have to be so lonely. Break your ideas into parts and delegate tasks. If a journal cut is in the plan, let the serials staff make suggestions as to which journals should go. They may know better than you which journals sit on the shelf and which are constantly asked for. Watch for signs of anger. Librarians and library staff like order and hate change. They will be very unhappy about doing things differently. If someone starts talking loudly, acting inappropriately around customers or administration, showing signs of resistance, taking numerous mental health days, don't ignore it. Talk to that person. If necessary, get human resources involved.

Use your staff's suggestions. If someone makes a good suggestion to improve on your plan, use it. You will be amazed at how quickly you will get buy-in from your staff if you actually use their ideas. Many "talk the talk" of listening to staff. Few "walk the walk." A good thing to do is make sure all the procedures and routines that don't change are emphasized. Every bit of order in the staff's lives should be reinforced.[2] If there is a Monday morning donut party every Monday at 8:00 a.m. then make sure the donuts show up at 8:00 a.m. Don't change anything that doesn't have to change.

Time your changes appropriately.[3] Making too many too fast will confuse your staff and your patrons and jeopardize their stability. Try to give your staff time to learn a new way of doing things before you change something else. Loudly tout the benefits of the new way over the old one. Inform your patrons of the new change so they are not confused when they come into the library. Remember, change takes patience, planning, and communication. If you do it right, everyone benefits. Start early to plan and initiate change. Be prepared to make changes in your changes.

OUTSOURCING

At some point in the process, outsourcing may seem attractive. Maybe, as I experienced during a downsizing, someone who is doing a vital job such as cataloging is leaving and an electronic catalog would be easier to maintain. Maybe you need to combine two jobs into one and there is still not enough work for one person. With all the changes in media production over the last few years, your media department may need to be examined. Are you paying someone to take photos for Web pages when digital cameras have taken over most of those duties? Do you have a slide producer (film recorder) sitting idle when everyone does their own PowerPoint? Look at the function and not the person in the function. It may feel very cold to you but it must be done for the survival of the organization.

Many hospitals are saving money by outsourcing their IT functions. You might wind up on a committee that outsources these functions. Another area that hospitals are looking at for possible outsourcing is human resources (HR). In both IT and human resources, companies are finding that the systems are so complex and the bar keeps being raised so high that it is impossible for a small local department to keep up. Librarians, with their advanced knowledge of computer systems, can be very helpful to administration in the outsourcing of IT functions. You may even want to assume some of their duties. Many hospital librarians do a lot of computer and Web training. There may be an instance where jobbing a service out might save a lot of money (although it has been shown that sometimes it is more cost-effective to do the service in-house). Outsourcing decisions should not only be based on cost saving but also on improved service to your customers.

What should you do before you ask for bids from companies? First, make sure your mission is not affected by outsourcing a specific function. You would not want to outsource information-providing or interlibrary loan if the turnaround time would not be within benchmarks. Remember, your customers come first.

Next, establish an outsourcing team to look at all the issues involved, both strategic and tactic. Outsourcing may save money in the short term, but will future developments mean rehiring staff and re-creating the department? Someone from finance should be on the committee. He or she can look at the overall financial picture and provide real numbers.[4]

You should do an in-depth analysis of how the person or department performs duties now with flowcharts to chart the relationships to other players. Then flowchart the proposed change and critique the difference. Someone on the committee should do a risk analysis to make sure the changes don't run you afoul of HIPAA (Health Insurance Portability and Accountability Act), JCAHO, and other accrediting boards and commissions. In the end, you should not willy-nilly decide to drop a service or a person and let someone else have the responsibility for it. As with downsizing, many attempts to outsource fail, costing the hospital thousands.

BACK TO SURVIVOR: *THE MERGE*

Somewhere in this process, you may have to merge with an external organization (as when two hospitals merge) or merge with another department in the hospital. In recent instances, hospital libraries have been merged with training and development and/or nursing education to create education departments for the entire hospital. This is the time to go back to the island and pick up some advice from our friends on *Survivor* because the game has just changed.

As on *Survivor,* the game changes when you merge. Different alliances and different players surface. You must move quickly to adapt. Suddenly you are sitting around a table with a group you have never seen before, reporting to a boss you do not know. If you get caught in an internal merge, there are many things to remember. Most important is to meet with the other players. This proactive step will establish you as a player. Read about the issues faced by your partners. You should be seen as someone who can deal with global hospital issues and not just library issues. In meetings with your new group, take a leadership role. You may now report to a director instead of a vice president. This occurs more and more in hospitals. Quickly make it known that you are aware of the issues he or she is facing and can help solve them. Even though it may not be library work as such, you are a manager and your contribution should always be toward making the hospital a better place. Many library managers have successfully contributed to managing other departments. Don't shy away from this task. You can either be a player when the dust settles on the merger or a subordinate. For your library, it is best not to be a subordinate but an equal partner. The more layers of administration you go through to get your voice heard, the less effective you will be in telling the library's story and getting the funding you need. Don't be voted out of the tribe!

RETRAINING STAFF

Staff need to be retrained for their new roles. Certain things will have to be done before you start retraining. Redraw the staff organization chart and rewrite procedural manuals. Train area specialists to train their staff (or in a small library do it yourself). Chances are you will be dealing with an older staff between forty and sixty years old. Today, 49 million Americans are age fifty-five and over. In the next four decades, that number will jump to 91 million.[5] Chances are some of those employees are yours.

Retraining is always a smart plan. As a library director, you are probably very familiar with teaching people how to use new technology. But your library staff, aging as most workforces are, may pose special problems to retraining. By retraining, you are recognizing that your older employees are some of your most loyal and hard-working. The myth that older workers cost companies more money in salary and in health insurances costs than younger employees should be done away with.[6] Their experience and increased productivity more than make up for their place on the employee pay scale.

How do you retrain older workers? Train them just as you train their younger colleagues, although you need to listen more. They will have bought into the old systems deeply and fully. They will have opinions and probably won't be shy about making those opinions heard. You will need to do a lot of selling to convince them the new method is better. They will have to make the switch to the new method emotionally. Build some rewards into the system or in some way recognize the achievements of the older staff in learning the new systems. There may be a problem with giving up a precious job. Some staff will mindlessly try to hold on to an old task. In some instances, put your foot down and say, "That is not necessary anymore." Once again you will have to ask why something is done. What purpose does the task service? Is the task a duplicate of another task? Sometimes we keep paper copies of stuff when the electronic copies are very secure. Go back to your mission and ask if the task fulfills it.

LAYOFFS:
BEWARE THE EXECUTIONER'S SONG

At some part in this process, you may have to tell good, hardworking staff that the hospital no longer has need for their services. This is not a fun thing. Many managers dread letting staff go. Here is a way to make it as palatable as possible.

As with all things in business, a plan is better than no plan at all. A committee should be formed to handle layoffs. The committee should include the vice president for that division, you as manager, a representative from human resources, and anyone else deemed necessary. Layoffs should be handled individually. Staff should be treated with the utmost respect. The vice president should start the meeting by reiterating that the staff member in question is a valued member of the organization. His or her individual achievements should be recognized if at all possible. The financial situation of the organization should be explained in as much detail as possible. The reasons for the employee's layoff should be detailed. The emphasis should always be on the position being eliminated, not the staff member. The human resources representative should detail the benefits that the employee is entitled to. The employee's direct manager should offer support. All the material discussed should be on paper and given to the staff member to review at a later date. An appointment with a representative in human resources should be made so that the employee has a chance to review the information and ask questions. Some employees need that extra push of looking an HR rep in the face before he or she will say anything. No matter how much advance warning the staff member has had, he or she will be in shock and won't remember much of what was said.

You have worked very hard and penetrated that inner circle of management, thus insulating yourself and most of your library from direct cuts. You have been put on some influential committees that will decide the fate of your colleagues in other departments. This is a time to be very careful. Some people drunk with the heady enthusiasm of power (first time) volunteer to assist in laying off staff. Don't do this. Never become an executioner. The bad news should always be given to staff as a group and upper management should take its share of the responsibility. Executioners are universally despised long after the downsizing is over. After the deeds are done, upper management does not support its henchman well. Anecdotally, there seems to be a high incidence of executioners leaving the organization when their services are no longer needed. The foul odor of being a cutter remains for a long time. Staff don't forget that you cut a friend.

At this point, you may be in shock yourself. Studies show that executioners are still affected by their actions ten years after the event. One cutter said, "We put all—there were blackboards, so we put all the names on the boards, and we just sat them, and I can remember, it gave me the creeps, there was this stunned silence, and we felt like it was the Vietnam Wall or something. We were upset, all of us . . . saying, 'Look what we are doing to all those people! Isn't there any other way? Why are we doing this?' It was horrible."[7] Part of the survivor syndrome that will be discussed in the final chapter is the guilt you may have from laying off people. It is a real problem that must be dealt with if you are going to move on. Seek counseling if you or friends or family notice a change in your behavior. Never tough it out. Don't be a stone. Stone cracks and eventually crumbles.

THE UH-OH FACTOR AND BACKPEDALING WITH STYLE

Due to the downsizing, you had to cut hours the library is open. You had to cut staff and your journal budget. The first week after everything settles down, a physician will come to you and ask, "Why weren't you open on Sunday? I need the library open on Sunday." Or someone will say, "You cut my favorite journal. We can't maintain our specialty at the hospital without that journal. Cut something else, but not that." Someone might say, "We loved that e-journal. Why did you cut it?" (Bet you wish you had looked at the usage numbers before you cut based on assumptions.) Finally, you get a call from a physician saying, "Why did you cut (insert name)? She is your best employee and she is the wife of a member of my practice. Cut someone else."

You will make mistakes during this time. Mistakes come in all shapes and sizes: foolish mistakes, careless mistakes, stupid mistakes, innocent mistakes, and mistakes in judgment.[8] Mistakes generally come when you try to do too much in too little time, assume too much without checking the facts, are too proud to ask for help, or are too stubborn to listen. Humans make mistakes and during a downsizing, you may be at your human(est). You will be confused and tired. That one goof may seem like the biggest issue in your life because that is where the noise and heat is coming from.

Step back a bit and realize that it is not as bad as you are making it. Fortunately, you still have the criteria you used to make your cuts. Your paperwork is in order. You have your charge from administration and the approvals for your plan. You have your ducks in a row. You have that small amount of extra money you cut to play with. That is your fudge factor. If possible, bring something back that is important. Do it with some fanfare.

The following are a few things to do if you find yourself backpedaling on a decision:

- *Admit you are wrong.* What a concept! Don't cover up. Sometimes just admitting you were wrong diffuses the issue. Make it better. If you didn't look at the numbers correctly and made the wrong decision, say, "I made the wrong decision."

- *Make a temporary solution to make your customer happy.* Ask, "What can I do to resolve this issue?" Keep records of the conversation if necessary. If his or her favorite journal was cut and it will take months to get it reinstated, maybe you could offer him or her the table of contents from another library and free interlibrary loan until the subscription starts coming in again. Don't make your customers suffer for your mistakes (with responsibility comes accountability).

- *Have a permanent solution in the wings with a date when it will happen.* Everyone promises to make changes, but few will commit to a date for the change to occur.

- *Sometimes the mistake is not the problem.* It is how you handle the mistake. (Would Nixon have had to resign if he hadn't tried to cover up the Watergate break-in?)

- *Learn from your mistake.* Analyze why your initiative failed so you don't make the same mistake again. Learn from history, instead of repeating it.

- *Move on and try harder.* Don't brood. Failure is a part of life.[9] Do not ignore an obvious mistake, deny a mistake exists, shift the blame for a mistake, or use a mistake to give up and quit trying. I did that once. I used a downsizing to cut a beloved program to spite an administration that would strip me of my staff. It eventually backfired. When you do things for the wrong reasons, it usually does.

This is going to be a difficult time for you. Administration is not in a good mood. They are taking flack from the press, their customers, the board, physicians, and staff. Your library staff are angry about the cuts and their missing friends (along with all the new work they have to do as several jobs are melded into one). They are having trouble performing tasks in a new way. Your customers may be very angry at a lack of services. You may be taking heat from many directions. Administration may doubt your judgment. They may not support you when confronted by strong opposition, leaving you dangling in the proverbial breeze. This may be the most dangerous time (next to the phony war period), when tempers flair and your favorite doctor reacts when he or she finds out his or her favorite journal was cut.

CONFLICT RESOLUTION

Chances are somewhere during this process you will need to resolve a conflict. Most people try to avoid conflicts. Many librarians are especially hesitant to deal with a head-on confrontation with an angry customer but just like everything else, if you understand conflict and plan for it, you will survive it, make your customers happier, and learn from the experience.

Your attitude may be the biggest problem. If you consider all conflict to be negative, then you may need a change of thinking. Conflict is a natural part of life. It is with us always and may be a change agent. Sometimes so much entropy exists in an organization that conflict is necessary to start change happening. Consider a new way of looking at conflict. Think of it as a call to understand competing, but not incompatible, preferences and values. Or, consider it a periodic occurrence in any relationship that can be channeled toward better performance or growth.[10] Conflict that is well managed can tap your creativity and problem-solving skills and those skills in your colleagues.

How will you deal with conflict? Do you have a plan?[11] Like any good health care professional, you need to do a "Bates Physical Examination" of the problem. Try to assess the history of the situation and the roles and power of the parties involved before getting involved yourself. Is this a chronic or acute problem? Will it affect other systems? Your staff, who usually are the ones who first report the conflict to you, should be coached in what to look for and what to report.

Many times, managers make poor decisions because they have poor information. It is recommended that a "feedback form" be developed and kept at the front desk so staff can write down the important information that you need to properly attack a conflict. Many times, managers hear that "someone" complained about "something" (e.g., the copier or the circulation policy). You do not know who complained, how to reach that person to talk about the issue, what he or she complained about, and what is needed to resolve the issue. Think of the other stakeholders involved in this issue. If a physician wants to take out something from the reference shelf that is vital to nursing, nursing should be involved in the decision. Develop a form to capture that data and you will find that it is easier to deal with the issue.

Once you know the players and the issues, you can assess if you have a policy or procedure that covers it. Do the hospital policies and procedures somehow cover the issue? Then you can deal with the players.

Along the way, you may be drawn into the conflict and some anger may be directed toward you (or you may lose your cool). You can counter this by being the one to set the tone. Keep smiling. Acknowledge the seriousness of the situation but keep the tone professional. Don't allow name-calling or inflammatory accusations to get in the way. Deal with the issues, not the personalities. Sometimes acknowledging your feelings and the feelings of the other combatants is a good start to diffusing the issue. You give away nothing by saying, "You seem very angry. Will that anger help resolve this issue?" This is a variation of the TV psychologist Dr. Phil's "How's that working for you?" It quickly makes people realize that their behavior is not helping them. I once used that tactic to stop a physician who was trashing his office in a fit of rage. The physician realized how bad he looked and stopped his improper behavior. He could not bear to concede the high moral ground to a mere librarian. By the end of the day, the physician had sheepishly returned to offer his apology. Realize that you will probably work with the combatants again, so you need to resolve the issue and diffuse the situation. Nothing is as frustrating as winning the battle and losing the war.

Consider what elements you are willing to change to resolve the situation. If one person is involved and a policy or procedure is to blame, is it worth changing a hospitalwide policy unless an egregious injustice is involved? It is always a good idea to try to restate the person's concerns.

Approach the situation from the areas of agreement, not the areas of disagreement. If you get the combatants to agree, they may make a habit of it. From there, you can begin to craft a sentence or two that will make that person or persons happy. Repeat that sentence back to the person. An example would be, "So you are saying that you need to use the book for longer than three weeks and that if I will let you check it out for a month, you will be satisfied?" Now you have a solution that is hopefully workable. Remember to restate the solution several times until you get agreement from all parties. Sending a copy of the conversation in the form of a memo is not a bad idea if you are dealing with a person who has a convenient memory loss every now and then.

Conflict has many faces. There is conflict between you and staff and conflict between you and administration. What if the worst possible scenario happens? What if you are the one let go in a downsizing? It could happen. You are not the only one who makes mistakes. Administration could make a big one and downsize you. You will have to deal with a myriad of issues. You must quickly get a new job to support your family and keep your career on track. Chapter 8 describes how to get in gear and get another job quickly.

Chapter 8

Surprise!
You Are the One Downsized

It's a recession when your neighbor loses his job; it's a depression when you lose yours.

Harry Truman

Ask not for whom the bell tolls . . .

John Donne

They made a mistake. You are asked to come to a meeting with your vice president, the head of human resources, and members of the downsizing committee (or you are asked to come to a meeting in the boardroom and you are the only manager or nonadministrative type invited). Recently, a laid-off employee told me about feeling completely blindsided. He thought the meeting was about a voluntary severance package, only to discover that he was the only line employee in the room. A line from an old Gordon Lightfoot song goes, "The old soldiers say in their crusty old way there are too many troops in this room." Old soldiers know about downsizings.

You think to yourself, "This is bad. This is really bad. I just attended a few of these and was on the other side of the table." You sit at the long, highly polished table and the vice president says, "(John/Jill) you are a valued member of this organization. That fact makes what I am going to say that much harder. I have known you for years and have always respected your work ethic and ability to innovate. Your solution to that cross network file transfer problem was brilliant. I still can't believe you solved it when IT couldn't." After that, it is all words.

You don't hear much of what is said after that. You just hear a few words. "Laid off. Employee pool. Severance package. Not you, it is the position we are eliminating. You are a great employee. This was necessary for the organization. It is all on the Net anyway." Those words keep coming back to haunt you. "It's all on the Net." You are in shock. You did everything right. You got the highest annual reviews that the organization can give. Your vice president praises you up and down the organization. Your talents and innovative skills are the stuff of legend in your hospital and the state. You are on national Medical Library Association committees, for Lord's sake. You are still laid off.

BENEFITS OF BEING LAID OFF

You are not alone. Over two-thirds of any group of people have been laid off at some time in their lives. You may be angry at the un-fairness of it. In an informal survey, about 82 percent of laid-off em-ployees said they were angry about their termination (the rest are just relieved).[1] Deal with it. Prospective employers can detect your anger at your former employer "like stale cigarette smoke on a wool suit." Like the smoke, it poisons the air all around (and employers worry about the secondhand smoke you will generate if hired. Will the smell linger? Are you a toxic employee?). A prospective employer hears the negative things you are saying and thinks, "If that is what he or she says about them, what will he or she say about us?" Alarm bells go off and red lights start flashing. The interview is very short and un-successful. You really didn't get a chance to describe what a great em-ployee you would be.

Talk to your friends.[2] Blow off steam with them and not in the in-terview. Many of them have been fired. They will be able to offer ad-vice. Talk particularly to the ones who have survived and thrived. They will tell you how they survived. They may offer coping strate-gies. Don't just talk to one friend. Talk to at least three and synthesize their advice, throwing out the kooky off-the-wall stuff. Don't spend too much time on revenge fantasies or "what I should have said" com-ments. Realize that it is time to move on and do so. Now that you real-ize there is hope, you can begin to plan to get that new job.

People who consider their layoff an opportunity and not the end of their life do better. They adjust better and get better new jobs. Maybe it is time to step back and gain a healthier sense of identity. Many people identify themselves too closely with their careers and consider their value based on their salary or title. Are you like that? Do you consider yourself a librarian first and a person second? Is it time to reassess your priorities? Through marriage, children, hobbies, church, friends, pets, and age, I have learned that work should be one shard in the mosaic that is the healthy individual. For harmony, all the glass shards should be about the same size and fit perfectly. If one shard is too large, all the other shards will not fit.

Being laid off will challenge you. It will expose you to new ideas and circumstances. (Try running through an airport at 10:00 p.m. at night trying to catch the last flight to your job interview, jumping turnstiles like O. J. in a Hertz commercial, having no idea where you will be sleeping the night before the interview, for stress and adventure.) You may find yourself in many situations out of your comfort zone. You may need to take a temporary job beneath your skill level. You may find that you can contribute at that level and derive satisfaction from a job well done even though you are no longer "the director" or hospital library information guru. A little humility is not a bad thing. Many medical librarians develop a bad case of hubris, catching the disease from physicians and administrators. When you finally get a job that meets your qualifications, the experiences out of your field may be invaluable (out-of-the-box thinking). Being on-the-line for a while, you get a different view, a kinder gentler view of the trials your staff deal with every day.

This is the perfect time to reinvent yourself. Analyze why you went into hospital library work in the first place. Are those core values that brought you to this type of work the same for you, or have you changed? This is as good a time as ever to ask yourself some questions. Was I really happy doing hospital library work? What specifics about the work didn't I like? Do I like working with demanding doctors? Do I like the high-powered pressure-cooker atmosphere? What specifics did I like (besides the free lunches)? Would an academic medical center be a better fit for me? Would a corporate environment suit me better? Do you want to take another job that you are unhappy doing? You could take a temporary job in an area that has always interested you and see if you like it better or even volunteer if the severance and your situation allow it. You can return to school to get new skills or upgrade your skills. This is the perfect time to advance in another direction career-wise. Have you had the idea for a business in the back of your mind for years but never had time to really bring it to fruition?[3] More and more librarians are becoming information vendors. Grab a copy of *Information Today* and scan the articles. These new entrepreneurs are making money and having fun doing what they love to do. They provide information. Could you negotiate with several small hospitals in your area to become a circuit rider librarian? Would you be good at going from one library to another providing necessary library services (and satisfying their JCAHO requirements at a bargain price)? Some librarians find this very rewarding. There is a new challenge every day.

Do you have a background in sales? Think! As a hospital librarian you know hundreds if not thousands of physicians and other health care personnel. Maybe your undergrad background is in biology or chemistry. You are a wiz at medical terminology and can quickly learn new scientific information. Become a pharmaceutical firm representative and sell those physicians a product, using your friendships with physicians that you have nurtured over the years to your advantage.

Look into the library, book, or electronic services markets for jobs. Library degrees are not just for librarians anymore. We are in the middle of the information age. That is an important paradigm to remember. Business and health information stopped being a nice thing to have and started being a commodity in the 1960s. As a hospital librarian, you have been in the middle of pushing the need for health information to health professionals for years.

Some librarians are taking their professional Web-writing skills and making money in the private sector. With their flair for organization, advanced Web experience, and creative talents, some librarians make extraordinary Web writers. Your PowerPoint skills may come in handy creating beautiful presentations for the PowerPoint challenged. Are there companies in your area that could use a techno-boost? Have you seen a really bad PowerPoint presentation lately? (Everyone has.) You could go to that company or person and offer to improve their PowerPoint for a fee. Could physicians at your hospital use your PowerPoint skills to improve their statewide or national presentations? Does your hospital have a media services department or have you been informally consulting on PowerPoint topics for years?

Have you embraced the technological revolution with pure gusto? Taken lots of outside or in-house courses on computer technology? Can you fix 'em better than the techs and never have to call IT? Do you relish the thought of an ailing PC so you can repair it? Do you know more about the network systems in your hospital than the IT staff? Maybe you would make a great systems administrator. Consider getting Microsoft certification in networks. Courses are held all over the country on a regular basis. Basically, if you can't beat 'em, maybe you should join 'em.

With the support of the severance package (and hopefully an understanding spouse), you may want to take the leap into business. It has been shown that downsizings create thousands of small businesses. Your local Small Business Association can help you find a mentor and maybe a small business loan. Don't forget to do a business plan.

THE SEVERANCE PACKAGE: NEGOTIATING THE BEST DEAL

The use of a severance package allows a company to maintain a positive public image by demonstrating fairness and concern for its employees.[4] But packages are getting less and less rich for the rank and file. By the second or third downsizing in the cycle, they can get downright skimpy. This trend is creeping into middle management. Sometimes management tries to tailor the administrative costs of the package as to reduce their overhead because administration can eat up 20 percent of the entire plan's costs.[5] Be wary of plans that seem cumbersome and are poorly rolled out.

One thing that HR will try to do at that first meeting is use your shock against you (once again, shock and awe was used in business a long time before it made the battlefield). They will give you paperwork to sign, agreements to initial, and forms to fill out. It may seem like more paperwork than when you bought your house (and more confusing). They would love to have your signature on any document that waives your rights to sue them under certain circumstances. Unless they tell you to sign then and there or be escorted out of the building (or are holding your children hostage), do not sign anything until you take it back to your office and read it carefully. Legally, you have twenty-one days to review the document. Better yet, if you have the opportunity, run it past an employee lawyer. It may be worth the price of an hour of a lawyer's time to make sure you get all you can. It could mean thousands of dollars in benefits coming your way.

Quiz your laid-off colleagues in the organization to see what kind of packages they were offered. If you find a discrepancy, bring it up at the negotiations with administration.[6] It is advisable to dig out the company health insurance policy and read it carefully for any information about what the health coverage is for terminated employees. Some plans cover you through the end of the quarter, even when you have been laid off two months before that. Does what they are offering you mesh with what the stated company policy is? Can you negotiate for the better of the two? If you do not know the ins and outs of the employee manual and all company policy documents, now is the time to bone up. Management may be counting on your lack of knowledge, shock, and confusion.

It is advisable to shoot for the moon. What are they going to do? Fire you? Rank the ten most important severance benefits you want then push hardest for the ones at the top of the list.[7] You could be shooting for the most money. The current standard is one week of severance pay for each year of service. Try to trade off a benefit such as outplacement services for more money, especially if you have good leads on another job. Explain to management why you are worth the extra money.

Health benefits may be a particular concern if it entails your family's health coverage and you expect a long job search. Once again, try for everything you can get. If you are close to retirement age, you could ask your employer to add a few years to your employment record so you will be able to qualify for early retirement. This is sometimes called a bridge benefit and is very common with some companies. One hospital I worked at offered such a good bridge benefit that two employees jumped at the chance to take it. Only problem was that was 40 percent of my staff at that time. If this happens to you, remember you don't get extra credit for cutting more than is asked for.

Nearly 68 percent of large companies offer their laid-off employees some kind of outplacement counseling.[8] In a small field such as hospital librarianship, this can be an invaluable "benie." It is usually capped at three to six months. If you haven't been in the job market in a while and are not used to working the library job boards, this could be an important service. Negotiate for as much outplacement service as possible.

Other items that should be on your wish list include office space with a computer and telephone and keeping your e-mail and voice mail activated. That way, you can job hunt without prospective employers knowing you are out of a job. For some reason, prospective employers like to think they are stealing you away from another company and think less of people who are laid off.

If your PDA, laptop, pager, etc., are a few years old, the hospital has already depreciated them, and they are probably not worth much to the organization but may be invaluable to you in conducting a job search and hitting the ground running at your next job. You won't get stuff if you don't ask. Remember to back up and save all relevant information on disk before your leave. Think of those wonderful PowerPoint presentations you designed and the articles you wrote for publication. Save all your proposals and grant applications.

Some companies even offer help with relocation expenses. The cost of relocating a household can easily run into many thousands of dollars. If your company is not located in a major metropolitan area, and they recruited you, you may want to ask about including this benie in the mix.

Don't forget to ask about consulting opportunities and contract work. Could your hospital use your expertise as a freelance searcher or trainer? Could you teach MEDLINE four times a year for a fee? Could you work with continuing education and charge a fee for a Grand Rounds lecture? Can you justify your literature search fee based on how many malpractice suits you would head off? Maybe a few friendly physicians or local medical societies could write a few letters emphasizing how important these services are to older physicians who are not computer literate. Can you do searches on a fee basis to satisfy JCAHO requirements? If you feel you could use the regulations and certifications that all hospitals are bound by, go for it. This is one reason that it is best to leave on good terms with the hospital.

Maybe your reputation is the most important thing to you. So, negotiate how your layoff will appear in the local press and how the recommendations will be worded. That layoff could become a "mutually agreed upon separation." Maybe they can word the announcement to show it was not a firing for cause and that you were an excellent employee (kind of building a recommendation into your layoff notice). Maybe you should write the recommendations beforehand, emphasizing your accomplishments so the important issues are covered when your boss sits down to write one for you.

This is not a time for timid behavior. Bend the rules as much as possible. If they say, "This is the policy," say, "Oh, yeah?" Talk about the extraordinary things you have done for the hospital and the money you have saved them. Talk about the personal financial obligations that you incurred predicated on a paycheck from the hospital (and with little warning that that paycheck would cease). Talk about any commitments you have signed obligating your library to provide services to other libraries (this is a good time to talk about how these obligations will be met through selling your services back to the hospital as a freelancer). This is the time for total candor. The gloves should come off.

Get tough. If you suspect your former employer is breaking the law somehow with the severance package or downsizing (not applying fair standards, violating the Americans with Disabilities Act), get an employment lawyer[9] and let him or her duke it out with management. Is upper management using the downsizing as an excuse to get rid of senior employees close to retirement age? Severance packages must abide by the the Worker Adjustment and Retraining Notification Act (WARN), Employee Retirement Income Security Act (ERISA), The Age Discrimination in Employment Act (ADEA), and several other federal laws. WARN applies to any profit or nonprofit company that has more than 100 employees. A threatened lawsuit may be an eye-opener for management.

When you come to an agreement with your former employer, write a letter to him or her outlining the terms of the agreement. Include a phrase at the end of the letter that states, "If I'm incorrect in any respect, please let me know immediately. If I don't hear from you, I presume you agree." These words could cover you very well in your future dealings with the company. It is amazing what gets said in a semiheated discussion. It is always a good idea to document the conversation and have administration sign off on it. It also stops a lot of "I think he or she said" stuff from happening.

FALLACIES OF DOWNSIZINGS

Beware of several fallacies here. One, your organization knows what it is doing and of course the first proposal is the best it can do.

This "knows what it is doing" argument is the easiest refuted. Who got your company into its present financial mess? Is it the same people who are trying to get out of the financial quagmire? And just how many downsizings has your organization done? If it is the first one, the company will be tentative and prone to make mistakes. Most companies stumble when doing their first downsizing. The argument about "this is the best offer" is also easily refuted. Many corporations tailor their severance packages due to special circumstances.

The second fallacy is that you are powerless and that upper management holds all the cards. You do have power. Their well-orchestrated downsizing could easily run aground if a few people got lawyers and found some reasons to sue. The board would not look favorably on bad publicity at this point. Probably some board members opposed the downsizing. Your goodwill during this process is extremely necessary for the downsizing to take place smoothly. Your hospital does not want bad publicity. The higher up you are on the food chain, the happier they may want to make you. (At one organization I worked at, the organization chart was referred to as the food chain because it involved large fish consuming small fish and large fish smelling blood in the water and attacking other wounded large fish.) It is doubtful they want to lose business due to bad press. They want this over with as quickly and cleanly as possible. Sometimes they are willing to pay.

The third fallacy is the timetable. You have x number of days to take the plan and leave. That is what it says in all the paperwork, so it must be true. This is not true. Cookie-cutter plans that have no flexibility are destined to fail. Management usually has some contingency money set aside but will not tell you about it unless you ask. If your library has an important deadline coming up that management doesn't know about or didn't plan for, bring this up and ask for an extension. A simple mention of "Gee, it doesn't seem to me to be a good idea to let me go before a JCAHO site visit" may get you a few more months extension.

I was in a similar position. I had staff that had to finish vital projects. The departing staff had to have time to train the remaining staff in their new duties. With vacations already set, there just was not enough time to train staff. I requested and received three-month extensions for some of these employees. Other managers said it couldn't be done. Upper management said it was impossible. It can be done.

Just make your case well. If, at the end of this project, you can't make your case very well, you haven't been trying.

Some companies actually offer what is called a "stay-on" bonus. If a project is important enough to them, they may offer a retention bonus. One company offered some techies 75 percent of their salary for the ten-month transition—plus the full severance pay.

WHAT TO DO AFTER YOU HAVE BEEN LAID OFF

Bet you wish you had updated your résumé. Can you hear your mom saying, "You should have done what the nice man said in Chapter 2"? Before you pack your mementos into a cardboard box, consider taking these steps. You should:

- Wipe all personal files off your office computer (or save the files to disk, then wipe them) and use a program such as Eraser to ensure the files are really gone. Many people don't realize that when files are deleted, they are not really deleted and can be recovered. If you don't want the next person who uses your computer or the strange computer tech that kept your PC up and running to know your personal business or financial information (credit card or bank account numbers), then make sure those disks are clean. On the paper side, make copies of every program you developed, every brochure you designed, every Web page you wrote, every good review you have ever received from your boss, every report you wrote, every thank-you you ever received, and every poster you created. All these things are tangible examples of your output and are great at interviews.
- Prepare a keyword searchable résumé.[10] Companies now use databases to store résumé information (not to mention the big job boards such as Monster.com). They scan the information in instead of keeping tons of paper in the office. Nearly 73 percent of recruiters are on the Internet searching for candidates every day using keyword searching. Are they going to find you? If you have the right words in your résumé, you will be found quickly in a search later.
- Don't send your résumé as an e-mail attachment unless you are specifically requested to.[11] Some company firewalls don't handle

attachments well and there is nothing nastier than a hospital's firewall. Can you say "HIPAA"? Knew you could.

- If the company wants your résumé in text format, cut and pasted into an e-mail, send the e-mail to yourself first so you can clean up the text, and put in line breaks to make it readable.
- Most résumés sent via e-mail are viewed on a very small monitor that does not display the entire page. So start your résumé with your major accomplishments or the bullet points you want the employer to remember. This is similar to the problem of Web writers who design incredible Web pages on 21-inch super monitors. The pages are then viewed on 15-inch monitors, where the art, skill, and content are lost.
- Remember that corporations delete stored résumés after about six months, so reapply if you have to. Don't assume your résumé will be there forever.
- Create a simple cover letter stating the jobs you are looking for, locations, and salary range. It is suggested you drop the salary range on letters that go directly to companies but keep it for placement services where it is an important feature in limiting or broadening their search.
- E-mail your résumé to every recruiting firm in your niche. If you have been out of the job searching game for a while, much is done with e-mail and job boards and less and less through newspapers and snail mail. Use all available technology to get your message out there quickly and efficiently.
- Now forget about the recruiters. You have done your part, give them time to do theirs. Confirm that the information has gotten to them, then let them do their job. They can either answer your telephone calls or work on getting you a job.
- Network like crazy. Don't stop going to meetings, seminars, etc. You will get stale and out of touch. Keep in touch with colleagues (but not too in touch). They may be a great source of rumors on recently opened jobs.
- Organize your life around your new job—finding a job.[12] Get up at the same time you got up when you were working. Eat and exercise on the same schedule, but spend all day everyday working the phones, the newspapers, the Internet to find that new job. If you stay focused you will stay sane and find the job you need.

THE RIGHT ATTITUDE

Case History No. 1

Recently, I spoke to a just-downsized nursing professor about her experience. She said, "I got a lot of perks out of the university when they let me go. I got library use for my PhD thesis that I plan to finish this summer. I got some great references. I got office use for the summer and some other nice things. They let me keep my laptop. I really didn't want to work anymore and they gave me a great package of benefits. With my skills, if I want a new job, I could have one in no time. I have kept up with my training and am very marketable as a clinician or a teacher. I will decompress for a few days, let them take me to a few luncheons, then move on. I will miss this place, but I'm ready." That professor has the right attitude. She got everything she possibly could out of the old organization, took stock of her skills, and is moving on to other challenges.

Case History No. 2

Another laid-off employee said, "I was really upset for a few days. I couldn't sleep. I obsessed about my layoff. All I could do was walk my dogs and go over it in my mind. I thought about what I did wrong. How could I have done things differently? Then I drew up a plan. I know there is going to be less and less need for my services (medical photography) in the future because digital cameras are everywhere now. So, I'm going back to school to become a nurse. The demand for nurses is incredible right now. I love helping people. With my severance package and some help, I could be an RN in two years. I have been stale for too long. I am looking forward to this."

Case History No. 3

On the other side of the coin, the following is an example of someone who felt the whisper of the ax and lived to tell about it. This librarian writes on MEDLIB: "Our department manager recently told me that I was retained, even though I had volunteered to be laid off, because of my breadth of knowledge and flexibility. I think that extra edge for breadth and flexibility applies to nonrelated skills and experience as well. My current job includes other health education duties and I believe I was hired partly because I had experience in other areas besides librarianship. I've just completed an MPH (master of public health) and I know that my organization feels that makes me even more valuable to them." What a great honest story. Sometimes that added extra, that job you take on that no one else wants, is all that stands between you and a pink slip.

Suddenly, you are planning your layoff shower (or your colleagues are). This is a new trend in going-away parties that is catching on with some corporations. Instead of the cake in the conference room snoozer, staff are invited to come with rolodex cards of possible contacts for the laid-off employee. They may also bring samples of killer résumés or boxes of high- quality résumé paper. The idea is to make this last time with colleagues productive and fun. It should be a time for staff and friends to be supportive and helpful, not somber and negative. Anyone who has ever been at an employee going-away gathering knows how awkward they can be as people shuffle around not knowing what to say or do. They sometimes have a funereal atmosphere about them.

THE INTERVIEW

Consider the three "Vs" of interviewing: visual (appearance), vocal (voice), and verbal (what you say). About 93 percent of a person's communication effectiveness is determined by nonverbal communication. A study showed that you have about thirty seconds to make a positive connection between yourself and the person interviewing you.[13] Your interviewer may be making many conclusions about you long before you open your mouth. First impressions are very important. Dress accordingly. Most corporations on the East Coast still like to see applicants in suits in conservative blue and gray. Brown is still considered questionable as a business color. Skirts should be not more than three inches above the knee. Suits should not be out of date, with lapels no more than three inches wide. Save the cartoon ties for your first day at your new job. Your interviewers might not share your love of Scooby-Doo. If you are going from an academic institution to a hospital environment, you may be going from very casual dress to a semiformal or formal look. Consider this before you go to the interview. A call to the interviewer's secretary might not be a bad idea to find out what others are wearing. Don't slouch during the interview. When you stand, make sure your shoulders are back and your head is held high. Your handshake should be firm and dry. Make eye contact as much as possible. Show energy and enthusiasm. Showing a little excitement about the new position could go a long way.

If the first words out of your mouth are that you hate your former employer, then that is what the interviewer will remember about you. Don't act like a victim, blaming everyone at your former job from the CEO to the janitor for your layoff. Take ownership of your part of it. Remember, you have dealt with that anger and gotten rid of that baggage. Remember the following on the topic of anger and your employer. Just as you did that Internet search to find out about your prospective employer, corporations are using the Internet to check up on you. Even simple search engines such as Google will allow you to go into the newsgroups and type a name and retrieve all the information in those files as far back as 1995. If you said something negative about your employer in 1995 on a discussion board, in the newsgroup or usenet groups, it may still be there, poisoning your chances for a great new job. The moral of this story is never say anything in writing you don't want people to know about.

The first thing out of your mouth at the interview should be your skills, your experience, and your enthusiasm for the opportunity they are offering you. Of course, you should have thoroughly researched the company or hospital you are interviewing at so you know what they do and how you can contribute to their continued success. A trip to the local public library to peruse the business reference books is not a bad idea. Also, a Google search of the company and a peek at their Web page couldn't hurt. Nothing kills a candidate's chances faster than when one says, "I'd love to work here. By the way, what do you do?" It becomes very tedious for an interviewer to tell ten prospective candidates about the company mission.

Try to save any discussion of your termination for later in the interview after they have gotten to know you and are familiar with your skills and personality. If your prospective employer shows any interest in you, that is the time to bring up the downsizing/merger/layoff or BCE.

Here is the best way to bring up the nasty topic. When the employer has demonstrated an interest in you, say "When you check my references, you will discover I was laid off due to a downsizing at my previous job. I received the highest possible performance reviews every year (here are copies). I was part of a general downsizing. Many good employees were let go. There is not much more to say about it. I am ready to move on and continue my successes in my field." Don't say much more. You have translated to your prospective employer that you are ready to move on. You have said that it was not a disciplinary termination.

A good point to remember is that your prospective employer is on trial just as much as you are. If an employer grills you on your firing/termination/layoff to the point that you are uncomfortable, then it may be a huge red flag that this may not be a good place to work. If you are not treated with respect during the interview process, then it does not bode well for your employment. Is there chemistry between you and your prospective boss? You may find during interview discussions that you disagree with him or her on censorship, acquisitions policies, flextime, and a host of other issues. He may be a rabid Boston Red Sox fan and when you put that autographed Derek Jeter baseball on your desk the first day, it may signal the beginning of the end. You may chuckle at this, but relations between employee and employer become strained over the strangest things sometimes. So many times someone will say, "I thought I would love my new job but it turns out my boss is a jerk." (Maybe it is not your boss who is the jerk.) Did you bother to interview your boss at your employee interview to find out his or her pluses and minuses? Did you write down those pluses and minuses and decide if you can live with them?

While you were researching the corporation, did you check the Internet for anything on your new boss (e.g., articles written or committees chaired)? If he or she thinks cataloging is the only true calling for a librarian and you feel reference is the only place for a librarian, you will disagree a lot. Do you know anyone in the organization who could give you a heads-up on the employer to eliminate any faux pas from your conversation before they happen?

Even if you are offered the job (and the pay is great), you may not be happy in the new position. A rule of thumb is, interview your employer about the job as hard as he or she interviews you. You should know certain facts about the job. Make a list of issues that are important to you. Writing down the answers will show you to be more interested in the position than someone who just sits "slack-jawed" for an hour in front of the interviewer.

Be careful during the interview and listen to what the interviewers say. I have been interviewing prospective employees for twenty-five years and been on the other side of the desk more times than I can remember. I have sat in on interviews during which another interviewer in the team turned to a prospective employee and said, "I see here that you are married with children. Will that stop you from doing your duties?" That person violated the Americans with Disabilities Act. If you are not sure what can and cannot be asked during an interview, get to your state employment agency and ask. They will most likely supply you with that information.

Another rule of thumb, don't mention benefits at the first interview. If you say something such as, "I want to work for your company because your retirement benefits are good," your prospective employer may assume that you will hang around for twenty years not doing much, waiting until you can collect retirement benefits.

Finally, prospective employers are looking at how you treat other employees during the interview period to see if you are a good fit with their company. Always be very cordial and professional with secretaries and administrative assistants. If a scheduling snafu occurs (and when there are a lot of applications, cancellations and errors are bound to occur), take it in stride even if you are freaking inside. Be as flexible as possible in scheduling an interview. Employers like to see flexibility and an employee who will work with them. If you have to fill out forms for human resources, be polite there, too. Not only will this help you get your new job, but making friends early helps you in your transition from "newbie" to part of the team.

Don't despair. You will find another job and survive this. The same analytic skills and cool head that kept you going and successful in the heavy-duty pressure-cooker atmosphere of the average hospital will help you thrive and survive your downsizing. I have never met a hospital librarian who wasn't intellectually tough on some level.

Because you are a winner, you will take what life hands you and make the best of it. Coming through to the other side, you will realize you are better for having survived the chaos and uncertainty. Remember, few great warriors are made during peacetime and few great presidents during times of peace and prosperity. The crucible of strife is necessary to refine greatness. Greatness comes from great challenges, and there is an upside to living in interesting times (paraphrasing the ancient Chinese curse).

Enough of this shameless cheerleading! If you are not downsized, many final lessons can be learned before you are ready to confront the beast.

Undefeatability lies with ourselves.

Sun Tzu

Chapter 9

When Hostilities Cease

What does not kill him makes him stronger.

Frederick Nietzsche

Nietzsche never went through a downsizing.

Michael J. Schott

AFTERMATH

As stated in the opening chapter, downsizings tend to fail at an alarming rate. Like suicide is described as a permanent solution to a temporary problem, downsizings can be knee-jerk, short-term solutions to long-term problems with the organization. A downsizing rarely leads to increased profitability and sometimes results in exactly the opposite. Two-thirds of the downsized corporations polled did not meet their projected revenues after the first year.[1] One analysis showed that the average stock performance after a corporate downsizing was 4 percent, while the performance for the S&P 500 during the comparable time period was a gain of 29.3 percent.[2]

Corporations are too timid in their cutting, or their projections are too optimistic. Staff or administration sabotage the process. Business cycles are not adequately predicted. The wrong people are downsized. Sometimes the corporate climate is so polluted by a sloppy downsizing that nondownsized staff leave. Since the best employees are the ones who can find jobs elsewhere the quickest, who will be left? Will the mediocre and disaffected be all that remains of a once fine staff?

Sometimes, too many people are downsized and even though the corporation is profitable, not enough people are available to handle the incoming new business.[3] Lines become long. Customers are unhappy. The organization's reputation starts to slip. Fewer people use the services, and another downsizing is necessary because profits are down again. Welcome to the vicious circle of life.

It is a slippery slope. As with a lion that develops a taste for human blood, the single downsizing leads to other downsizings. The lion is difficult if not impossible to sate. You can expect two or three downsizings, usually in two- to three-year cycles. It is best if you take a little time to grieve, lick your wounds, and then plan for the next round, even if the next round is not in sight. You hear the lion's roar before you see him. Be ready.

ALTERNATIVES TO DOWNSIZING

There are alternatives to downsizings. Costs can be reduced without layoffs. Did you know that eighty of the Fortune 100 Best Companies to Work For in 2002 had no layoffs in 2001?[4] Is it because these great-to-work-for companies are smart, caring, and thus very successful? Is it because the employees work hard for these companies, and they know that a layoff is a last resort, not a first resort? Do these companies see their employees as expenses or assets? Most likely, they see their employees as valuable assets, treat them accordingly, and are thus rewarded with superior work and loyalty. It is emphasized at those companies that a downsizing with layoffs is the last option, never the first. Restructuring is a word that is bandied about during a downsizing. Management usually uses this term to mean a layoff, but there are different kinds of restructurings. Perhaps nonprofitable areas of the hospital must be made profitable or eliminated and the personnel sent to areas that are profitable and booming. Sometimes, nonprofitable outpatient facilities must be closed. It takes a big management team to say they made a mistake and deal with just that issue before it jeopardizes the entire bottom line. It takes a big management team to cut from the head down and not the bottom up. Consider the old adage, "Bottlenecks start at the top."

Once I worked at a hospital that bought a laundry and dry cleaner (not exactly their core business). The only plus from this turned out to be discounted dry cleaning for employees. After years of not turning a profit, they sold it. Certain kinds of downsizings do work. If a company is selling off unprofitable assets and that is the reason for cutting people, then that cutting could lead to greater profitability.[5] Regrettably, this is seldom the case with a not-for-profit hospital or academic medical center. Sometimes the mission gets in the way. If cardiology is losing money but the hospital has the only angioplasty services in a hundred miles, then cardiology must stay if the hospital is to fulfill its mission.

To stave off a downsizing, staff can be cross-trained and thus moved from one position to another in case someone leaves through retirement or voluntary separation. A flexible staff can do much more than one that is locked into a specific job. People are paid for the job they are doing, not the job they used to do. Best of all, they have a job. This is one thing a hospital library can do successfully: cross-train staff within the department and find other areas of the hospital to cross-train with. Share duties as much as possible. Cover for vacations and illnesses.[6]

Once I found myself transporting patients during a time when transporting was down several employees and a hiring freeze was on. (Able-bodied men in administration were asked to be volunteer transporters.) I was none the worse for wear from the experience. I actually got the chance to talk to patients and learned the internal workings of several departments as never before. I learned to properly move a patient from the bed to a wheelchair or gurney. I learned what steps to take when transporting a very contagious patient to limit my exposure to pathogens. Since medical records and transporting were under the same department, I learned to file medical records. I also learned to appreciate some of the unsung heroes that make up a hospital (e.g., the transporters, the radiologists, and the nursing staff). Some of these people were the most patient teachers I have ever met. It is also very good personal PR (marketing yourself). Two years later, when the call went out for volunteer transporters, I was the first in line. You are seen as a person who will chip in and work when the going gets tough.

Some or all staff can take a cut in hours worked; thus, everyone suffers instead of a few. This has proved successful for some companies, although it may not work in health care where some staff are already in very short supply.

Some companies don't overhire. Being fiscally responsible, they just have the employees they need to have.[7] This is called "rightsizing" (as opposed to rightsizing by downsizing). It is also called "just-in-time hiring." This could be considered the human resources equivalent of "just-in-time purchasing." Temporary staff can be used instead of hiring new permanent personnel. Those companies work lean and smart and don't downsize.

Some companies are noted for their active retraining programs.[8] They are smart enough to recognize change before it comes and retrain their staff for necessary jobs. When the paradigm shifts, the employees are moved into new roles instead of being laid off. In these organizations, staff loyalty is very high and turnover is low, thus saving training dollars for new employees.

SURVIVOR SYNDROME

According to a 1995 survey of 681 hospitals, poor morale due to layoffs is by far the worst human resources problem in the health care industry.[9] Administration expects survivors to be grateful they were spared and to quickly forgive what happened to their colleagues. They may expect you to put your feelings aside and work harder (fewer people means more work for those who are left). Employees, on the other hand, may feel anger toward management or show their discontent through mumbled griping, negative attitudes, and even hostile outbursts. Prepare to be disliked. For the first time, your staff may actually turn against you, not understanding why you had to do what you did. If someone is laid off, you, being nearby, may bear the brunt of their displeasure. If an employee's hours are cut, you may have to work with that angry person for a long time.

It is never easy after a downsizing, especially one that has not been handled well. Many organizations fail to do their homework and communicate to staff that they are valued members of the work team. They fail to communicate that everything possible was done before the final alternative of downsizing was initiated. Increased workload occurs as several jobs are melded into one. (Sometimes this, too, is handled poorly.) The new organization may have smaller or tighter salary increases and reduced benefits (thus affecting families). There may be a great deal of organizational uncertainty. There is probably much less career-oriented training and development.

After the downsizing, you or your staff may:

- feel a loss of control leading to denial of responsibility;
- feel that there has been injustice, thus breeding resentment;
- feel bitterness or make excuses; and/or
- take your feelings out on co-workers, families, or patients.[10]

In other words, you may have survivor syndrome. If untreated, survivor syndrome leads to a set of attitudes, feelings, and perceptions that encompass anger, fear, distrust, guilt, and severe cynicism. You may be wary of taking any risks at work. You do the minimum to just get by. Without risk-taking, there is no possibility of achievement. You may have a lack of commitment to your job. New ideas just don't come. The "why bother" syndrome is in full bloom.

What to do if you or your staff suffer from this debilitating illness? Some suggestions are:

- Take some time to mourn the loss of your colleagues who were downsized. The loss of these colleagues can be as painful as the death of a loved one. A little closure is not a bad thing. Take a fallen friend to lunch.
- Do not work more than fifty hours a week. A downsizing is an exhausting occurrence both mentally and physically.
- Organize your life.
- Sleep at least six hours each night.
- Eat correctly and take a vitamin supplement. High stress consumes some vitamins.
- Take fifteen minutes each day to meditate or pray, or both.
- Leisure read.
- Do thirty minutes per day of aerobic exercise.
- Make a conscious effort to perform one act of kindness a day.
- Work on your sense of humor.
- Know that this will pass (try to be optimistic).[11]

Treat staff and all others fairly and justly. People want "it" to be all over. If you have no new information, give them hope and direction by emphasizing the importance of what we do. Tell them the work goes on, that they are valuable members of the organization, and that their work makes a difference at their institution. This can help defuse the "us versus them" syndrome where staff view management as the enemy. Even when staff cannot be loyal to the institution, they can be loyal to patients and their other customers. Survivor syndrome responds to vigorous intervention just as many septic diseases do. Take a cue from physicians and meet it head on and conquer it.

It cannot be overemphasized that survivor syndrome must be dealt with in yourself and in others. Recently a library director confided to me that he had to lay off several employees in a department other than the library because of budgetary shortfalls in the organization. Later he heard that someone on his staff was calling the laid-off employees and telling them that the library director was personally responsible for the layoffs and that they were all "payback firings." This was completely untrue. The library director used a strict set of criteria to base his assumptions on and remained within administration guidelines at all times. He said he couldn't believe his own staff was working against him after all he had done to keep their jobs. His staff had become "toxic." It will take a great deal of time and effort to detoxify them. Remember what was stated earlier in the book. People do bizarre things under stress. That incident was documented. The document was sent to HR and upper management. The employee responsible was shown to have a history of this type of behavior and was dealt with by upper management.

DODOS:
A CAUTIONARY TALE OF THE FUTURE

The professor said, "Consider the walleye pike." Simon settled back in his comfortable educhair in his living room to listen to another long semipointless analogy. "In the twentieth century, scientists put walleye pike in an aquarium separated in half by clear glass. In the other half of the aquarium, small fish were placed. The pike could see the food fish through the glass. They bumped into the clear glass again and again trying to get to the food. Eventually they gave up. The glass was removed. The pike believed that the separation was still there and that the food fish were unobtainable even though the fish swam around them. The pike starved to death. Can anyone tell me why? And yes Simon, this will be on the final."

"Jennifer, do you know why?" The pretty blonde holostudent said after thinking for a moment, "Because the pike didn't believe they could get the fish?" "Jennifer, that is the obvious answer. Didn't you access the assigned Web data?" Jennifer started to stammer. Simon accessed the controls on his couch, did an illegal personal message to Jennifer, and whispered to her, "There was a paradigm change." "There was a paradigm change?" she said. "Yes. Good, Jennifer. There was a paradigm change. The pike died because they did not understand the beneficial change that occurred. They could have feasted and lived but didn't because they could not recognize change or deal with change. It is extremely important to recognize change and plan for it."

Simon looked around his room. He was comfortable sitting at home listening to and responding to the holographic image of the professor. The teacher had substance and in all ways looked like his real image. He could see holographic images of the other students in his class. He could interact with them and debate with them. They had substance, as his image had to them.

Simon thought again how superior it was to go to college in the twenty-second century, when college came to you as much as the other way around. Cheap electronics and the Internet+2 had made going to school as easy as paying the money and telling the homenet what the coordinates are for the lecture. And this was one of the more interesting courses: Technological Change and Career Obsolescence in the Twentieth-Century or as students liked to call it, Dodo 101. It is a must for anyone going into global corporate finance. Although the professor did a lot of old-style lecturing instead of putting you into holographic re-creations of actual events and grading your response. If you don't understand what is going on, how can you profit from it?

Simon was glad the first lecture on buggy whip manufacturers of the early twentieth century was over and the professor was getting to the meat of the course. The professor's booming voice woke Simon out of his reverie. "Consider the hospital librarian." Simon licked his lips and settled back in his chair. The professor was known for excoriating professions that died because of their own stupidity, and hospital librarians were a pet peeve of the professor. Simon wondered if there might be a medical librarian in the professor's ancestry. He would have to do a quick ancestry search on the professor after class. That would be delicious if it were true. It would be like having a horse thief in the family.

"In the nineteen-sixties, there were few medical librarians except at the very largest institutions. By their heyday in the late nineteen-eighties, there were thousands upon thousands of hospital librarians." With a flick of the professor's wrist, a line graph floated in the air before the students showing a dramatic rise in the number of medical librarians. "Tiny hospitals with less than eighty-five beds had hospital librarians. Why? What changed to make these people valuable in a health care setting?"

Several people buzzed the professor at once and as usual the ones who knew how to use the controls on their couch, probably from interacting with holographic vidgames, were able to buzz first. "Thomas, yes?" "The information explosion that started in the nineteen-sixties," Thomas answered. "Partially correct, Thomas. Anyone else? Remember organisms such as businesses and corporations survive because of profitability and self-interest. Follow the money. Where is the money in this case? What was happening in medical information in the nineteen-sixties, nineteen-seventies, and nineteen-eighties?" Jennifer answered, "It was exploding exponentially. No one could keep up." "Good, Jennifer, very good. No one could keep up. And remember your data dumps. What happened for the first time in the nineteen-sixties to medical information?" "It became a commodity?" someone called out. "Excellent. It became a commodity. There was so much of it and it was so hard to manage in paper form that it became a commodity. This was the time of the first information vendors like Dialog, BRS, and of course, MEDLINE."

"Let's review the facts." The professor said, "Play program A900B6." Behind him on an electronic supersmart board, images from that bygone era flashed by. The images showed student physicians from the 1960s thumbing through *Cumulated Index Medicus* volumes. Then librarians using dumb terminals and acoustic couplers to access MEDLINE. Then personal IBM computers were used. Then CD-ROM MEDLINE discs were shown being used. Finally the Internet(1) was displayed. The students were fascinated with the old archaic machinery from a bygone era. It was like watching Alexander Graham Bell use the telephone.

"When MEDLINE came into existence and people had to pay to access the medical literature instead of using the paper *Index Medicus,* medical librarians suddenly began to appear in medical libraries. Why? Because MEDLINE cost sixty dollars an hour to search. A capable, properly trained medical librarian could find the answer to a query in a few minutes and cost a few dollars. A poorly trained novice searcher could spend hours and hundreds of dollars finding the same answer. Think of the cost to a hospital of having a physician spend an hour of his or her day trying to find an answer to a medical problem instead of seeing patients. It was so cost inefficient as to be laughable.

"So there was an economic advantage to having qualified medical librarians. They prospered. Every hospital had one." Charts and statistics appeared in the air by magic showing the increase in MLA membership per year. "They organized paper collections and kept staff aware of new developments in medicine. They taught, trained, assisted in hundreds of ways. In some hospitals in the early nineteen-eighties, the only personal computers that could be found were in the library. Medical librarians pioneered the use of CD-ROM based databases, ten years before they became popular. They were truly the knowledge managers of their organizations, demonstrating new software, assisting with IT functions, running media departments and auditoriums. Some librarians were the original IT departments in their hospitals. Some pioneered networking in their respective institutions. Many pioneered the Internet, the Web, and consumer health information. There are instances where the medical librarian was the originator of the hospital's Web page. It was a golden age."

The professor spoke again. "Then two things happened. One professional, one technological. Those medical librarians did nothing to assure their continuance. They had professional societies. They had standards. But they failed to convince the powers that be to set those standards in stone. They climbed the mountain but failed to plant a flag. They could have lobbied for their expansion and survival. They could have demanded tougher standards. Their self-marketing was nonexistent. A very important fact to remember is always market your profession. If you are not fighting for yourselves, no one else will. A few tried to buck the appeasement that went on in the profession. These visionaries were pulled down by the appeasers, who were afraid to speak up and tell others about the vital role they played in their hospitals. The standards were so watered-down as to be of no help at all.

"When the first paradigm hit, no one was ready and like a wave the medical librarians were swept away." A hand immediately shot up. "Professor what was this paradigm that doomed these librarians?" "What happened in nineteen-ninety-seven in medical information? Can anyone answer Ted's question? No? Simply, they made MED-

LINE, the rock upon which medical librarians stood, free." There was a stunned silence.

"Yes, the paradigm changed. MEDLINE was free to all and easy to use. Suddenly there was no need for medical librarians. They did a poor job of articulating what they did and why. By the year twenty-ten, there were fifty percent fewer medical librarians than there were in nineteen-eighty. When the shortsighted hospital downsizings came about, the medical librarians, considered nonprofitable support staff, were the first to go. By twenty-fifty, there were literally none. A few of the best survived and did quite well as independent information providers."

"Some of their companies are on the New New York Stock Exchange. I hear that stock on the new exchange is trading at ten and up. Rebounding nicely after the crash. The sad thing was it did not have to be. Medical librarians performed many vital functions in hospital libraries. They supported teaching and education. In some hospitals, they were in charge of continuing medical education. Even though MEDLINE was free and easy to use, few physicians could use it properly. Medical librarians with their unique training could find important answers in minutes that would take others hours.

"The rise of the first Internet only made this situation worse. There was more and more information. Some of this information was false or misleading. Yet no one in the hospital had the unique job of making sense of the health information explosion. Only now with advanced probability computers can we estimate the number of malpractice lawsuits that they averted by supplying medical information to physicians when needed. The number is equal to the gross national product of the world and satellite systems. For so little investment, hospitals got so much and never knew it."

A hand went up. "Professor, so what? Why do we care what happened to an obsolete bunch of dodos?"

"You are being redundant, Carly. Dodo and obsolete are the same in this case. But the reason is quite clear to anyone who has studied business trends of the early twenty-first century. What was the most important thing that happened in twenty-thirty?" Twenty hands immediately went up. "You all know that it was the bankruptcy of the old United States brought on by the health malpractice crisis in twenty-twenty-five." The holographic hands went down. "Let's review, because this is a very important concept to understand.

"Physicians in the United States were being sued for malpractice at an alarming rate. Although technologically advanced as no nation had ever been, health care in the United States lagged behind most industrial nations. Physicians' groups were continually going out on strike. Students would not go into health care because of these problems. The profession was too expensive and too volatile. More and more physicians retired. People could not get health care or pay for it when they could find it.

"I know that one of my colleagues traces the fall of health care in the United States to the arrival of what he calls 'B-school thugs' in the nineteen-seventies and nineteen-eighties. Although they kidnapped health care and created a huge overpaid management level that siphoned off precious resources, they were only partially to blame. A strong healthy nation became a poor sickly one. There were not enough healthy people left to maintain vital functions such as defense or policing the streets. Water treatment systems started to collapse. Meat was not inspected. A sickly United States was susceptible to attack from any tin-pot third world dictator. The new diseases of the new millennium did not help. AIDS-6 and Northwest Nile Virus wiped out a tenth of our population and overwhelmed an already fragile health care system. The national treasury went broke paying for Medicare and Medicaid. The crisis became so bad that President Chelsea Clinton tried to nationalize health care as her mother tried to do years before. But, it was too little too late. At least she blocked the multinational pharmaceutical companies from buying the United States and turning it into a giant chemical plant like northern New Jersey.

"The nation went bankrupt and we had to become a territory of Canada to survive. The United States went from the greatest nation on earth to a territory without voting rights in the space of fifty years."

"What could have been done and what do the medical librarians have to do with this?" a student asked. "I am glad you asked. Look at this holomap of the old United States. See the states where the ratio of medical librarians to physicians is high. Connecticut is a good example. Notice their lack of malpractice suits. Now look at states such as West Virginia. Notice the complete lack of medical librarians in relation to the physician population. Notice that no one was there to keep physicians informed as to new advances in medicine. Now notice the high incidence of malpractice suits that bankrupted the state and drove good doctors out of the state to greener pastures. What can we conclude?"

A student chimed in, "That states with a high rate of medical librarians had lower instances of malpractice suits because physicians used these resources to practice state-of-the-art medicine. Smart doctors went to states with good health information resources, and good information resources kept the doctors smart." "Exactly! An A for this course, Rich. Someone once wrote, 'For want of a nail, the shoe is lost; for want of a shoe, the horse is lost; and for want of a horse, the rider is lost.' Thus, for lack of medical librarians effectively providing health information to physicians and nurses, that beautiful experiment of the United States was lost.

"Tomorrow we will juxtapose this discussion with a discussion of the rise of the computer technician in the same environment. How is it that these machine geeks went from the back room inserting punch cards into huge machines to the boardroom commanding huge institutions? Why did the knowledge managers, the medical librarians, fall so low and these machine operators become vice presidents? It is a fascinating study in how not to become a dodo. You can do a data dump from 123.330.4405.5 and access the pertinent information before class tomorrow." A groan is heard from the class. "Any questions? Then that will be all. End program."

Simon's holographic screen went blank except for some text reminder of the reading assignments. He thought to himself, "Have to prepare for the test in three-D Web writing two-o-one. The cybermath in that class is a killer."[12]

Note

The previous tale details that downsizings at this time in history are dangerous to hospital librarians. The very future of our profession is being jeopardized by short-sighted decisions by administrators and weak response by hospital librarians. Every librarian should fight hard to keep library jobs in hospitals and health care in general. Every loss should be mourned, every success celebrated. We make a difference in our hospitals. We must stand up and say this from the highest point in our institutions, whether it is the boardroom or the CEO's office. We must initiate studies in our profession that continually prove our worth. We must fight any weakening of the standards. We must initiate public relations campaigns that tell the public our value, so that they demand medical librarians like they are being persuaded to demand qualified nurses. If we don't, no one else will. If we fail, it is no one's fault but our own.

CONCLUSION

Finally, it is recommended that career self-management is an antidote for survivor syndrome. If you can reclaim your work life and feel in control of the situation, you will survive whether you are downsized or a survivor. Your organization may have shown casual disregard for you or your staff. They may have shown some near-criminal behavior. Will you be comfortable working for these people? Will you feel the same? Now is a good time to imagine what you want to be doing (if you did not do this in Chapter 2). If you still feel that your library and hospital are the place for you, stay. Prosper. Enjoy. If you feel that this incident has changed the way you perceive your organization negatively and the feelings don't go away, get help. If there is still no change, find another job where you can reclaim your spirit.

If you have gone through a downsizing, you have just gone through one of the most traumatic events that can occur in your life. It is right up there with divorce or the death of a loved one. People need time to heal. Smart people know when they need help and they get it. A psychologist told me, "You don't take on a tank with a feather duster and you don't deal with severe psychological trauma by ignoring it." I have learned that you don't stand alone and unprepared against events that shake your world to their very foundation. Only a fool stands alone.

"If"
by Rudyard Kipling

If you can dream—and not make dreams your master;
If you can think—and not make thoughts your aim;
If you can meet with Triumph and Disaster
And treat those two impostors just the same;
If you can talk with crowds and keep your virtue,
Or walk with Kings—nor lose the common touch,

If neither foes nor loving friends can hurt you,
If all men count with you, but none too much;
If you can fill the unforgiving minute
With sixty seconds' worth of distance run—
Yours is the Earth and everything that's in it,
And—which is more—you'll be a Man, my son.

Notes

Chapter 1

1. Schott, Michael. "Corporate Downsizing and the Special Library (Getting Tired of Lemons)." *MLA News* (April 1996): 1, 6-7.
2. Peters, Thomas J. *In Search of Excellence* [videorecording]. Washington, DC: PBS Video, 1985.
3. Corporation. Investorwords.com. Available at <www.investorwords.com/cgi-bin/getword.cgi?1140>.
4. Rondeau, Kent V. and Wagar, Terry H. "Managing the Workforce Reduction: Hospital CEOs Perceptions of Organizational Dysfunction." *Journal of Healthcare Management* 47(May-June 2002): 161.
5. "Wayne Cascio Is Down on Downsizing." *Across the Board* 39(November/December 2002): 13.
6. What is a paradigm shift? Available at <http://www.taketheleap.com/define.html>.
7. Toffler, Alvin. *Future Shock*. New York: Random House, 1970, p. 14.
8. Wallace, Cynthia. "Medicare Spending Cuts Are Set at $2.77 Billion in Proposed '86 Budget." *Modern Healthcare* 15(January 4, 1985): 22.
9. Monahan, Catherine. "Surviving Staff Reductions." *Clinical Leadership and Management Review* 15(March/April 2001): 130.
10. Young, Susan and Brown, Hazel N. "Effects of Hospital Downsizing on Surviving Staff." *Nursing Economics* 16(September-October 1998): 258.
11. Bellandi, Deanna. "The Quiet Restructuring: Blaming Feds, Hospitals Shed Workers, Facilities in Droves." *Modern Healthcare* 28(December 14, 1998): 2.
12. Tully, Patricia and Saint-Pierre, Etienne. "Downsizing Canada's Hospitals, 1986/1987 to 1994/1995." *Health Reports* 8(Spring 1997): 33.
13. King, David N. "The Contributions of Hospital Library Information Services to Clinical Care: A Study in Eight Hospitals." *Bulletin of the Medical Library Association* 75(October 1987): 291.
14. *The Downsizing of America*. New York: Times Books, 1996, p. 4.
15. Lurie, Jonathan. Downsizing. Princeton University. Available at <www.geocities.com/WallStreet/Exchanger/4280>.
16. Young and Brown. "Effects of Hospital Downsizing," p. 258.
17. Ibid., p. 259.
18. Ibid., p. 258.
19. Averill, James. "Health Care Reform and Hospital Downsizing: Facing New Realities." *Hospitals and Health Networks* 67(December 20, 1993): 8.
20. Nelson, Bob. "The Care of the Un-downsized." *Public Management* 80(April 1998): 20.

Chapter 2

1. Grossman, Frank. "Updating Your Personal Balance Sheet (Also Known As Your Resume)." *AFP Exchange* 23(March/April 2003): 82.

2. Smith, Gregory P. "Creating the Perfect Resume." *Career World* 31(November/December 2002): 19.

3. Goleman, Daniel, Boyatzis, Richard, and McKee, Annie. "Primal Leadership." *Harvard Business Review* 79(December 2001): 44.

4. Ibid.

5. Drohan, William W. "Writing a Mission Statement: How to Capture the Essence of Your Association in a Well-Written Statement." *Association Management* 51(January 1999): 1.

6. Ibid.

7. Ibid.

8. Wuorio, Jeff. What Makes a Good Boss? MSN Business. Available at <www.bcentral.com/articles/wuorio/131.asp?cobrand=msnandLID=3880>.

9. Ibid.

10. Ibid.

11. Gluck, Jeannine and Hassig, Robin Ackley. "Raising the Bar: The Importance of Hospital Library Standards in the Continuing Medical Education Accreditation Process." *Bulletin of the Medical Library Association* 89(July 2001): 272.

12. McGowan, Jessie. "For Expert Literature Searching, Call a Librarian." *CMAJ* 165 (November 13, 2001): 1301-1302.

13. Klein, M.S., Ross, F.V., Adams, D.L., and Gilbert, C.M. "Effect of Online Literature Searching on Length of Stay and Patient Care Costs." *Academic Medicine* 69(June 1994): 489-495.

14. Homan, J. Michael. "The Role of Medical Librarians in Reducing Medical Errors." *HealthLeaders Online.* Available at <www.healthleaders.com/news/feature1.php?contentid=38058>.

15. Marshall, J.G. "The Impact of the Hospital Library on Clinical Decision Making: The Rochester Study." *Bulletin of the Medical Library Association,* 80 (April 1992): 169.

16. King D.N. "The Contribution of Hospital Library Information Services to Clinical Care: A Study in Eight Hospitals." *Bulletin of the Medical Library Association* 75(October 1987): 298.

17. Lindberg, D.A., Siegal, E.R., Rapp, B.A., Wallingford, K.T., and Wilson, S.R. "Use of MEDLINE by Physicians for Clinical Problem Solving." *JAMA* 269(June 23-30, 1993): 3129.

18. Schacher, L.F. "Current Clinical Issues: Clinical Librarianship: Its Value in Medical Care." *Annals of Internal Medicine* 134(April 17, 2001): 717.

19. Palmer, R.A. "The Hospital Library Is Crucial to Quality Healthcare." *Hospital Topics* 69(Summer 1991): 20-25.

20. Hammond, Patricia and Priddy, Margy. "Hospital Libraries Are an Economically Sound Investment." *MLA News* 341(November/December 2001): 1.

21. Baldwin, Jerry. "Mn/DOT Library Accomplishments." *Transport Connect.* Available at <www.transportconnect.net/top.html>.

22. Byrne, Tina. "Supposedly Free Online Content Contains Hidden Costs for Firms." *Houston Business Journal*. Available at <www.houston.bizjournals.com/houston/stories/2003/03/24/fpcus5.html>.

23. Ibid.

Chapter 3

1. Tiffan, William R. "Health Care Downsizing: A Survival Guide." *Physician Executive* 21(September 1995): 22.

2. Ibid., p. 23.

3. Ibid.

4. Daniels, Cora. "Tuesday, Bloody Tuesday." *Fortune* 141(March 6, 2000): 418.

5. Ibid.

6. Eison, Paul and Reitz, Victoria. "Consultants: The Roots of All Evil?" *Machine Design* 74(March 21, 2002): 96.

7. Parmenter, David. "A Consultant's Advice on How to Get the Most from Consultants." *New Zealand Management* 50(May 2003): 50.

8. Eison and Reitz, "Consultants," p. 96.

9. Ibid.

10. "Communicating Better at Work." *Library Personnel News* 13(Spring/Summer 2000): 10.

11. Ibid.

Chapter 4

1. The Phony War: October 1939-April 1940. World War II Multimedia Database. Available at <www.worldwar2database.com/html/phonywar.htm>.

2. "Sick of Downsizing." *IIE Solutions* 32(July 2000): 66.

3. McGarvey, Robert. "Dealing with a Downturn." Entrepeneur.com. Available at <www.entrepreneur.com/Your_Business/YB_SegArticle/0,4621,289067—,00.html>.

4. Ibid.

5. Shrader, Ralph W. "The Inner Circle." *Executive Excellence* 19(December 2002): 20.

6. Ibid.

7. Ibid.

8. Ibid.

9. Karasik, Paul. "The One-Minute Position." *On Wall Street* 12(September 2002): 94.

10. Ibid.

Chapter 5

1. Davidoff, F. and Florance, V. "The Informationist: A New Health Profession?" *Annals of Internal Medicine* 132(June 20, 2000): 996.

2. OCLC Library and Information Center Report. *Five-Year Information Format Trends*. OCLC March 2003.

3. Ibid.

4. Ibid.

5. Ibid.

6. Ibid.

7. Emmerich, Roxanne. "What's in a Vision?" *CMA Management* 75(November 2001): 10.

8. Ibid.

9. Collett, Stacy. "SWOT Analysis." *Computerworld* 33(July 19, 1999): 58.

10. Ibid.

Chapter 6

1. The Guide: SUNY Geneseo's Online Writing Guide. Available at <www.writingguide.geneseo.edu/goodwrite.shtml>.

2. Ibid.

3. "The Basics of Good Writing." AIT Extension Language Center. Available at <www.languages.ait.ac.th/EL21NITG.HTM>.

4. Raibert, Marc H. "Good Writing." Available at <www.alice.org/Randy/raibert.htm>.

5. Sloboda, Brian. "Creating Effective PowerPoint Presentations." *Management Quarterly* 44(Spring 2003): 20.

6. Endicott, Jim. "Visual Aids—Using Visual Aids Effectively—Visuals Aren't Everything." Presenters University. Available at <www.presentersuniversity.com/courses/show_vausing.cfm?RecordID=313>.

7. Sloboda, "Creating Effective PowerPoint Presentations," p. 22.

8. Raibert, "Good Writing."

9. Endicott, "Visual Aids."

10. Neuborne, Ellen. "Top Four PowerPoint Gaffes." *Sales and Marketing Management* 155(June 2003): 22.

11. Sloboda, "Creating Effective PowerPoint Presentations." p. 25.

12. Wild, Russell. "PowerPoint Overkill." *Financial Planning* 33(July 2003): 74.

13. Venus, Matt and Takher, Arjum. "Presentations." *Student BMJ* 9(December 2001): 463.

14. Ibid.

15. Ibid.

16. Ibid.

17. Sherman, Rob. "10 Presentation Skills Top Executives Live By." *Business Credit* 104(June 2002): 46.

Chapter 7

1. Rosner, Bob. Resisting change. ABCNEWS.COM Working Wounded. Available at <www.abcnews.go.com/sections/business/WorkingWounded/WORKING WOUNDED.html>.

2. Johnson, Lorie and Kaplan, Bonnie. "10 Ways to Make Change Easier to Accept." *Nursing87* 17(October 1987): 32X.

3. Ibid.

4. Flannery, Thomas P. and Heckathorn, Larry. "How to Build Your Business Case for Outsourcing." *Benefits Quarterly* 19(Third Quarter 2003): 8.

5. Bove, Robert. "Retraining the Older Worker." *Training and Development* 41(March 1987): 77.

6. Ibid., p. 78.

7. Wright, Barry and Barling, Julian. "The Executioner's Song: Listening to Downsizers Reflect on Their Experiences." *Canadian Journal of Administrative Sciences* 15(December 1998): 341.

8. Ramsey, Robert D. "The Art of Making Mistakes." *Supervision* 64(January 2003): 7-9.

9. Ibid., p. 10.

10. Siders, Cathie T. and Ashenbrener, Carol A. "Conflict Management Checklist: A Diagnostic Tool for Assessing Conflict in Organizations." *Physician Executive* 25(July/August 1999): 32.

11. Blackard, Kirk. "Assessing Workplace Conflict Resolution Options." *Dispute Resolution Journal* 56(February/April 2001): 58.

Chapter 8

1. Bolles, Richard N. "How to Deal with Being Fired." JobHuntersBible.com. Available at <www.jobhuntersbible.com/library/hunters/fired.shtml>.

2. Ibid.

3. Montgomery, Tara. "Benefits to Being Laid Off." Laid off in Silicon Valley. Available at <www.laidoffinsv.com/laid_off_benefits.html>.

4. "Severance: The Rules Have Changed." *HR Focus* 80(March 2003): 1.

5. May, Douglas H. and Brandenburger, Tom. "Controlling the Cost of Severance." *Financial Executive* 19(January/February 2003): 20.

6. Alderman, Lesley. "Walk Out the Door with All the Money You Deserve." *Money* 25(August 1996): 66.

7. Ibid., p. 68.

8. "7 Immediate Steps After Being Laid Off." Jobs.net. Available at <www.jobs.net/resources/candidates/job_search/7_steps_after_layoff.html>.

9. Alderman, "Walk Out the Door," p. 68.

10. Ibid.

11. Ibid.

12. "How to Survive Being Laid Off." Third Age. Available at <www.thirdage.com/news/archive/ALT04010214-02.html?hvnav>.

13. Martin, Carole. "The 2-Minute Drill." MSN Careers. Available at <editorial.careers.msn.com/articles/twominutedrill/>.

Chapter 9

1. Nelson, Bob. "The Care of the Undownsized." *Public Management* 80(April 1998): 21.

2. Reh, F. John. "Alternatives to Layoffs." Available at <www.management. about.com/library/weekly/aa070901.htm>.

3. "Wayne Cascio Is Down on Downsizing." *Across the Board* 39(November/December 2002): 14.

4. Ibid.

5. Ibid.

6. "How No Layoffs Can Work." *Business Week Online.* Available at <Web23. epnet.com/citation.asp?tb=1and_ug=dbs+1+1n+en%2Dus+sid+85B11BB1%2D19>.

7. Ibid.

8. Bove, Robert. "Retraining the Older Worker." *Training and Development Journal* 41(March 1987): 77.

9. Ciancio, Jack. "Survivor's Syndrome." *Nursing Management* 31(May 2000): 44.

10. Curtin, Leah. "Editorial Opinion: Surviving 'Survivor Syndrome.'" *Nursing Management* 27(October 1996): 7.

11. Ibid., p. 8.

12. Schott, Michael J. "Dodos 101." *Journal of Hospital Librarianship* (accepted for publication).

Bibliography

BOOKS

Adams, Scott. *Dilbert and the Way of the Weasel.* New York: Harper Business, 2002.

Conrad, Barnaby and Schulz, Monte, eds. *Snoopy's Guide to the Writing Life.* Cincinnati, OH: Writer's Digest Books, 2002.

The Downsizing of America. New York: New York Times Books, 1996.

Florida, Richard. *The Rise of the Creative Class.* New York: Basic Books, 2002.

Giuliani, Rudolph and Kurson, Ken. *Leadership.* New York: Hyperion, 2002.

Kuhn, Thomas. *The Structure of Scientific Revolution.* Chicago: University of Chicago Press, 1970.

McKee, Martin and Healy, Judith, eds. *Hospitals in a Changing Europe.* Philadelphia: Open University Press, 2002.

Peters, Thomas T. and Waterman, Robert H. *In Search of Excellence.* New York: Warner Books, 1984.

Rifkin, Jeremy. *The End of Work: The Decline of the Global Workforce and the Dawn of the Post-Market Era.* New York: Putnam Books, 1995.

Shaara, Michael. *The Killer Angels.* New York: McKay, 1974.

Toffler, Alvin. *Future Shock.* New York: Random House, 1970.

Torre, Joe. *Ground Rules for Winners: 12 Keys to Managing Team Players, Tough Bosses, Setbacks, and Success.* New York: Hyperion, 1999.

JOURNALS

Abrams, Stephen K. "Are You Building Your Library with the Right Stuff?" *Computers in Libraries* 19(September 1999): 76-80.

Aiken, Linda H., Clarke, Sean P., and Sloane, Douglas M. "Hospital Restructuring: Does It Adversely Affect Care and Outcomes?" *Journal of Health and Human Services Administration* 23(Spring 2001): 416-442.

Alderman, Lesley. "Walk Out the Door with the Money You Deserve." *Money* 25(August 1996): 66-68.

Averill, James. "Health Care Reform and Hospital Downsizing: Facing New Realities." *Hospitals and Health Networks* 67(December 20, 1993): 8-40.

Ball, Rafael. "Future Trends in Special Library Services." *Inspel* 34(3/4) (2000): 133.

Bean, Daria L. "Training Your Staff and Yourself to Communicate Effectively." *National Underwriter* (Life and Health/Financial Services Edition) 106(March 18, 2002): 11-12.

Bellandi, Deanna. "The Quiet Restructuring: Blaming Feds, Hospitals Shed Workers, Facilities in Droves." *Modern Healthcare* 28(December 14, 1998): 2-4.

Berry, John N. "Inventing the Library Future." *Library Journal* 126(September 15, 2001): 6.

Blackard, Kirk. "Assessing Workplace Conflict Resolution Options." *Dispute Resolution Journal* 56(February/April 2001): 57-62.

Bove, Robert. "Retraining the Older Worker: Interest Rises in Keeping the Older Worker in the Workplace." *Training and Development Journal* 41(March 1987): 77-78.

Bright, Lauren and Jacobs, Jerald A., eds. "Giving Staff Advance Notice of Large Layoffs." *Association Management* 54(October 2002): 21-22.

Bunyan, Linda E. "Tai Chi and the Art of Downsizing." *National Network* 25(October 2000): 6-7.

Burke, Ronald J. "Hospital Restructuring and Downsizing: Taking Stock: A Symposium, Part 1." *Journal of Health and Human Services Administration* 23 (Spring 2001): 381-387.

Ciancio, Jack. "Survivor's Syndrome: When Restructuring Means Layoffs, Prepare for the Psychological Impact on Employees Who Stay." *Nursing Management* 31(May 2000): 31, 43-45.

Collett, Stacy. "SWOT Analysis." *Computerworld* 33(29)(July 19, 1999): 58.

"Communicating Better at Work." *Library Personnel News* 13(Spring/Summer 2000): 3.

Cullen, Lisa Takeuchi. "Where Did Everyone Go?" *Time* 160(November 18, 2002): 64-66.

Curtin, Leah L. "Editorial Opinion: Surviving 'Survivor Syndrome.'" *Nursing Management* 27(October 1996): 7-8.

Daniels, Cora. "Tuesday, Bloody Tuesday." *Fortune* 141(March 6, 2000): 418.

Davidoff, F. and Florance, V. "The Informationist: A New Health Profession?" *Annals of Internal Medicine* 132(June 20, 2000): 996-998.

Dougherty, Richard M. "Planning for New Library Futures." *Library Journal* 127(May 15, 2002): 38-41.

Drohan, William M. "Writing a Mission Statement: How to Capture the Essence of Your Association in a Well-Written Statement." *Association Management* 51 (January 1999): 1.

Dube, Monte. "Restructuring Public Hospital to Meet Marketplace Demands." *Healthcare Financial Management* 50(February 1996): 38-40.

Ehrenhalt, Alan. "In Search of a World-Class Mission Statement." *Governing* 10(March 1997): 7-8.

Eison, Paul and Reitz, Victoria. "Consultants: The Roots of all Evil?" *Machine Design* 74(March 21, 2002): 96-97.

Emmerich, Roxanne. "What's in a Vision?" *CMA Management* 75(8) (2001): 10.

Fisher, Anne. "Surviving the Downturn." *Fortune* 143(April 2, 2001): 98-104.

Flannery, Thomas P. and Heckathorn, Larry. "How to Build Your Business Case for Outsourcing." *Benefits Quarterly* (Third Quarter 2003): 7.

Florian, Ellen. "Layoff Count." *Fortune* 143(May 14, 2001): 38.

Gluck, J.C., Hassig, R.A., Balogh, L., Bandy, M., Doyle, J.D., Kronenfeld, M.R., Lindner, K.L., Murray, K., Peterson, J., and Rand, D. C. "Standards for Hospital Libraries 2002." *Journal of the Medical Library Association* 90(October 2002): 565.

Gluck, Jeannine C. and Hassig, Robin A. "Raising the Bar: The Importance of Hospital Library Standards in the Continuing Medical Education Accreditation Process." *Bulletin of the Medical Library Association* 89(July 2001): 272.

Goleman, Daniel, Boyatzis, Richard, and McKee, Annie. "Primal Leadership: The Hidden Driver of Great Performance." *Harvard Business Review* 79(December 2001): 42-51.

Greenglass, Ester R. and Burke, Ronald J. "Stress and the Effects of Hospital Restructuring in Nurses." *Canadian Journal of Nursing Research* 33(September 2001): 93-108.

Grossman, Frank. "Updating Your Personal Balance Sheet (Also Known As Your Resume)." *AFP Exchange* 23(March/April 2003): 82.

Hammond, Patricia A. and Priddy, Margy. "Hospital Libraries Are an Economically Sound Investment." *MLA News* 341(November/December 2001): 1.

"How 'No Layoffs' Can Work." *Business Week Online* (November 6, 2001): 1.

Johnson, Lorie and Kaplan, Bonnie. "10 Ways to Make Change Easier to Accept." *Nursing87* 17(October 1987): 32X.

Karasik, Paul. "The One-Minute Position." *On Wall Street* 12(September 2002): 94.

Kaye, Beverly, L. "The Kept-On Workplace." *Training and Development* 52 (March 98): 32-38.

Kilpatrick, Anne Osbourne, "When in Doubt, Don't: Alternatives to Downsizing." *Management* 2(1999): 209-219.

King, David N. "The Contribution of Hospital Library Information Services to Clinical Care: A Study in Eight Hospitals." *Bulletin of the Medical Library Association* 75(October 1987): 291-301.

Klein, M.S., Ross, F.V., Adams, D.L., and Gilbert, C.M. "Effect of Online Literature Searching on Length of Stay and Patient Care Costs." *Academic Medicine* 69(June 1994): 489-495.

Lindberg, D.A., Siegel, E.R., Rapp, B.A., Wallingford, K.T., and Wilson, S.R. "Use of MEDLINE by Physicians for Clinical Problem Solving." *JAMA* 269(June 23/30, 1993): 3124-3129.

Lisoski, Ed. "Four Ways to Do More and More with Less and Less." *Supervision* 59(August 1998): 3-6.

Lowe, Frank. "Positioning to Prevail in a Merger or Acquisition." *AFP Exchange* 23(March/April 2003): 96.

Maharana, Bulu and Panada, Krushna Chandra. "Planning Business Process Re-engineering (BPR) in Academic Libraries." *Malaysian Journal of Library and Information Science* 6(July 2001): 105-111.

Marshall, Joanne G. "The Impact of the Hospital Library on Clinical Decision Making: The Rochester Study." *Bulletin of the Medical Library Association* 80(April 1992): 169-178.

Mastering Mission and Vision Statements. *Association Management* (January 2002): 25.

May, Douglas H. and Brandenburger, Tom. "Controlling the Cost of Severance." *Financial Executive* 19(January/February 2003): 20.

McManus, Kevin. "Your Mission (Must You Accept It?)." *IIE Solutions* 32(June 2000): 20-21.

Monahan, Catherine. "As We See It: Surviving Staff Reductions." *Clinical Leadership and Management Review* 15(March/April 2001): 130-132.

Nelson, Bob. "The Care of the Undownsized." *Public Management* 80(April 1998): 20-22.

Neuborne, Ellen. "Top Four PowerPoint Gaffes." *Sales and Marketing Management* 155(June 2003): 22.

Palmer, Raymond, A. "The Hospital Library Is Crucial to Quality Healthcare." *Hospital Topics* 69(Summer 1991): 20-25.

Parameter, David. "A Consultant's Advice on How to Get the Most from Consultants." *New Zealand Management* 50(May 2003): 50-56.

Piturro, Marlene. "Alternatives to Downsizing." *Management Review* 88(October 1999): 37-42.

"Preparing a Vision Statement." *Futurist* 36(July/August 2002): 59.

"Public Speaking: Overcoming the Jitters." *Nursing 2002* 32(January 2002): 68.

Ramsey, Robert D. "The Art of Making Mistakes." *Supervision* 64(January 2003): 7-10.

Resnick, R. "IRB and You, the Hospital Librarian." *National Network* 26(October 2001): 5, 8.

Ritchey, David and Turner, Dudley B. "The Public Relations of Layoffs." *Public Relations Quarterly* 46(Summer 2001): 32-36.

Roling, Judy. "The Top 10 Strategies for Dealing with Redesign or Resizing." *Journal of Trauma Nursing* 4(January-March 1997): 12.

Romaine, Steve. "If Consultants Misdirect You, Maybe It's Because You Allow Them To." *American Banker* 168(April 11, 2003): 6.

Rondeau, Kent V. and Wagar, Terry H. "Managing the Consequences of Hospital Cutbacks: The Role of Workforce Reduction Practices." *Journal of Health and Human Services Administration* 23(Spring 2001): 443-469.

Rondeau, Kent V. and Wagar, Terry H. "Managing the Workforce Reduction: Hospital CEO's Perceptions of Organizational Dysfunction." *Journal of Healthcare Management* 47(May-June 2002): 161-176.

Rondeau, Kent V. and Wagar, Terry H. "Reducing the Hospital Workforce: What is the Role of Human Resource Management Practices?" *Hospital Topics* 80(Winter 2002): 12.

Schacher, Loraine. "Clinical Librarianship: Its Value in Medical Care." *Annals of Internal Medicine* 134(April 17, 2001): 717-726.

Schott, Michael J. "Corporate Downsizing and the Special Library (Getting Tired of Lemons)." *MLA News* (April 1996): 1, 6-7.

Schott, Michael J. "Dodos 101." *Journal of Hospital Librarianship* (accepted for publication).

Serb, Chris. "Is Remaking the Hospital Making Money?" *Hospitals and Health Networks* 72(July 20, 1998): 32-33.

"Severance: The Rules Have Changed." *HR Focus* 80(March 2003): 1, 11, 13-14.

Sherman, Rob. "10 Presentation Skills Top Executives Live By." *Business Credit* 104(June 2002): 46-47.

Shrader, Ralph W. "The Inner Circle." *Executive Excellence* 19(December 2002): 20.

"Sick of Downsizing." *IIE Solutions* 32(July 2000): 66.

Siders, Cathie T. and Aschenbrener, Carol A. "Conflict Management Checklist: A Diagnostic Tool for Assessing Conflict in Organizations." *Physician Executive,* 25(July/August 1999): 32-37.

Sloboda, Brian. "Creating Effective PowerPoint Presentations." *Management Quarterly* 44(Spring, 2003): 20-34.

Smith, Gregory P. "Creating the Perfect Resume." *Career World* 31(November/December 2002): 18-20.

Snyder, Gerald. "Communicate Positive Attitude to Staff." *DVM* 33(May 2002): 70-71.

Talone, Patricia. "A Values-Guided Downsizing." *Health Progress* 83(March-April 1983): 39-42.

Tennant, Roy. "The Engines of Innovation." *Library Journal* 127(June 15, 2002): 28-30.

Thomas, Robyn and Dunkerley, David. "Careering Downwards? Middle Managers' Experiences in the Downsized Organization." *British Journal of Management* 10(June 1999): 157-169.

Tiffan, William R. "Health Care Downsizing: A Survival Guide.*" Physician Executive* 21(September 1995): 22-23

Tully, Patricia and Saint-Pierre, Etienne. "Downsizing Canada's Hospitals, 1986/87 to 1994/95." *Health Reports* 8(Spring 1997): 33-39.

Venus, Matt and Takher, Arjum. "Presentations." *Student BMJ* 9(December 2001): 463.

"Wayne Cascio Is Down on Downsizing." *Across the Board* 39(November/December 2002): 13-14.

Wild, Russell. "PowerPoint Overkill." *Financial Planning* 33(July 2003): 74-75.

Wright, Barry and Barling, Julian. "The Executioners' Song: Listening to Downsizers Reflect on their Experiences." *Canadian Journal of Administrative Sciences* 15(December 1998): 339-354.

Yallof, Jesse and Morgan, Curt. "Beyond Performance Standards: How to Get the Most from Your Outsourcing Relationship." *Benefits Quarterly* 19(Third Quarter, 2003): 17-22.

Young, Susan and Brown, Hazel N. "Effects of Hospital Downsizing on Surviving Staff." *Nursing Economics* 16(September-October 1998): 258-262.

Zimmerman, Eilene. "Why Deep Layoffs Hurt Long-Term Recovery." *Workforce* 80(November 2001): 48-53.

ELECTRONIC RESOURCES

Baldwin, Jerry. Mn/DOT Library Accomplishments. Available at <www.transport connect.net/trupdate/article2_main.html>.

Bolles, Richard N. How to Deal with Being Fired. JobHuntersBible.com. Available at <www.jobhuntersbible.com/library/hunters/fired.shtml>.

Byrne, Tina. Supposedly Free Online Content Contains Hidden Costs for Firms. Houston Business Journal. Available at <houston.bizjournals.com/houston/stories/2003/03/24/focus5.html>.

Do You Have an Effective E-resume? JobsInMA.com. Available at <www.jobsinma.com/mis/page.asp?pagenum=410>.

Downsizing: More Than Just Losing a Job. Available at <www.1clark.edu/!soan 221/97/Downsizing.html>.

Endicott, Jim. Visual Aids—Using Visual Aids—Visuals Aren't Everything. Presenters University. Available at <www.presentersuniversity.com/visuals_Visuals_Arent_Everything.php>.

Geary, Leslie. Here Come the "Duppies." CNNMONEY. Available at <www.money.cnn.com/2003/06/12/pf/saving/duppies>.

The Guide: SUNY Genoseo's Online Writing Guide. Available at <writingguide.geneseo.edu/goodwrite.shtml>.

Gurney, Darrell. 7 Immediate Steps After Being Laid Off. Jobs.net. Available at <www.jobs.net/resources/candidates/jbb_serach/7_steps_after_layoff.html>.

Heathfield, Susan M. Survivors Can Soar After Downsizing. What You Need to Know About Human Resources. Available at <humanresources.about.com/library/weekly/aa012201a.htm>.

Hickok, Thomas A. Downsizing and Organizational Culture. Public Administration and Management: A Interactive Journal. Available at <www.pamij.com/Hickok.html>.

Homan, Michael J. The Role of Medical Librarians in Reducing Medical Errors. HealthLeaders Online. Available at <www.healthleaders.com/news/feature1.php?contentid= 38058andCE_Session=b80cd2372>.

Hornestay, David. Reconsidering Downsizing. *Government Executive Magazine.* Available at <www.govexec.com/reinvent/downsize/0796view.htm>.

How to Survive Being Laid Off. ThirdAge—Money Newsletter. Available at <www.thirdAge. com/news/archive/ALT04010214-02.html?hnav>.

Making Sense of Corporate Downsizing. Center for the Study of Alternative Futures. Available at <http://csaf.org/politics/downsize.htm>.

Martin, Carole. Ten Fashion Blunders: What Not to Wear to the Interview. MSN Careers. Available at <editorial.careers.msn.com/articles/whattowear/>.

Martin, Carole. The Two-Minute Drill. MSN Careers. Available at <editorial.careers. msn.com/articles/twominutedrill>.

McGarvey, Robert. Dealing with Downturn. *Entrepreneur Magazine.* Available at <www.entrepreneur.com/Your_Business/YB_SegArticle/0,4621,289067-1---,00. html>.

Montgomery, Tara. Benefits of Being Laid Off? Laid Off in Silicon Valley. Available at <www.laidoffinsv.com/laid_off_benefits.html>.

Myers, Margaret. Downsizing the Hospitals. *The Michigan Daily Online.* Available at <www.pub.umich.edu/daily/1996/may/05-29-96/news/news9.html>.

The Phony War October 1939-April 1940. World War II Multimedia Database. Available at <www.worldwar2database.com/html/phonywar.htm>.

Raibert, Marc H. Good Writing. Available at <www.alice.org/Randy/raibert.htm>.

Reh, John. Alternatives to layoffs. What You Need to Know about Management. Available at <management.about.com/library/weekly/aa070901.htm>.

Rosner, Bob. Working Wounded. ABCNews. Available at <abcnews.go.com/sections/ business/WorkingWounded/WORKINGWOUNDED.html>.

Rosner, Bob, Halcrow, Allan, and Levins, Alan. People Skills: How to Screen Out the Jerks in the Job Interview. ABCNews. Available at <abcnews.go.com/sections/ business/CornerOffice/CORNEROFFICE.html>.

What Is a Paradigm Shift? Available at <www.taketheleap.com/define.html>.

Writing Up Research: The Basics of Good Writing. AIT Extension Language Center. Available at <languages.ait.ac.th/EL21NITG.HTM>.

Wuorio, Jeff. Keynote Like a Pro: The Do's and Don'ts of Public Speaking. Business 2.0. Available at <www.business2.com/articles/mag0,1640,47799,00.html? cnn=yes>.

Wuorio, Jeff. What Makes a Good Boss? MSN Business. Available at <www. bcentral.com/articles/wuorio/131.asp?cobrand=msnandLID=3800>.

UNPUBLISHED REPORT

OCLC Library and Information Center Report. *Five-year Information Format Trends.* March 2003.

SYMPOSIUM

George, Jerry. CLIR What Users Are Telling Us. Symposium on Library Studies. CLIR ISSUES, May/June 2003.

DISSERTATION

Lurie, Jonathan. Downsizing. (Princeton University). Available at <www.geocities.com/WallStreeet/Exchange/4280>.

VIDEORECORDING

Peters, Thomas J. *In Search of Excellence.* Washington, DC: PBS Video, 1985.

Index

Across-the-board budget cut, 10-11
Adams, Scott, 18, 65
Age Discrimination in Employment
    Act (ADEA), 112
Arcari, Ralph, 33
Art of War (Tzu), 3
ArXiv, 70-71

Bad corporate event (BCE)
    across-the-board budget cut, 10-11
    buyout, 12
    consolidation, 12
    downsizing, 11
    dumbsizing, 11
    merger, 12
    reengineering, 11-12
    reorganization, 11-12
    restructuring, 11-12
    rightsizing, 11
    severance package, 12
    stealth downsizing, 11
Balanced Budget Act of 1997, 6
Baldwin, Jerry, 33
BCE. *See* Bad corporate event (BCE)
Benchmarks, 29-30
Budgeting, 76-78
Business model, 61-62
Business plan, 67
    budgeting in new millennium, 76-78
    case histories, 78-81
    considering options, 78-81
    SWOT-ing your organization, 73-75
    trends in libraries, 68-71
    vision statement, 71-72
Buyout, 12

Case histories
    being downsized, 116-117
    business plan, 78-81
    Phony War syndrome (PWS), 58-60
    presentation, 91-92
Certifications, 25-27
Chief information officer (CIO), 34-35
Chief knowledge officer (CKO), 35
Collins, Phil, 17
Conflict resolution, 102-104
Consolidation, 12
Consultants, 45-47
Continuing medical education credits
    (CMEs), 25
"The Contribution of Hospital Library
    Information Services to
    Clinical Care: A Study in
    Eight Hospitals" (King),
    31-32
"Corporate Downsizing and the Special
    Library (Getting Tired of
    Lemons)" (Schott), 2
Corporate paranoia, 40-41
Corporations
    hospitals as, 4
    view of downsizing, 4-5
"Current Clinical Issues: Clinical
    Librarianship: Its Value in
    Medical Care" (Schacher), 32

Dilbert (cartoon character), 5
Dilbert and the Way of the Weasel
    (Adams), 18, 65
Donne, John, 105

Downsizing
  aftermath, 121-122
  alternatives, 122-124
  announcement, 39
    communicating with staff, 47-49
    consultants, 45-47
    important points to remember
      during, 52-53
    library staff as tribe, 49-53
    paranoia, 40-41
    presentation, 43-45
    process, 41-42
    timing, 43
  business plan, 67
    budgeting in new millennium,
      76-78
    considering options, 78-81
    SWOT-ing your organization,
      73-75
    trends in libraries, 68-71
    vision statement, 71-72
  cautionary tale of future, 126-133
  corporate view, 4-5
  definitions, 13
    across-the-board budget cut, 10-11
    buyout, 12
    consolidation, 12
    dumbsizing, 11
    merger, 12
    reengineering, 11-12
    reorganization, 11-12
    restructuring, 11-12
    rightsizing, 11
    severance package, 12
    stealth downsizing, 11
  failure of, 13-15
  figures related to, 9-10
  health care reality, 6-9
  of hospital librarian, 105
    benefits of being laid off, 106-109
    case histories, 116-117
    fallacies, 112-114
    interviews, 117-120
    procedures after a layoff,
      114-115
    severance package, 109-112

Downsizing *(continued)*
  implementation of plan
    backpedaling, 100-101
    change, 93-95
    conflict resolution, 102-104
    layoffs, 98-99
    mergers, 96-97
    outsourcing, 95-96
    retraining staff, 97-98
    uh-oh factor, 100-101
  paradigm shift, 1-4, 5-6
  Phony War syndrome (PWS)
    business model, 61-62
    case histories, 58-60
    explained, 55-58
    inner circle and positioning,
      62-66
    opportunities from other
      librarians, 60-61
    recognizing opportunities, 58
  preparing for, 17
    advertising successes, 36-38
    benchmarks, 29-30
    certifications and regulations,
      25-27
    evaluation surveys, 29-30
    fiscal studies, 27-29
    flowcharts, 29-30
    intelligence-gathering, 35-36
    leadership, 20-21
    literature, 30-34
    management style, 24
    mission statement, 21-24
    need for libraries, 34-35
    organizational charts, 29-30
    résumé, 18-20
  presentation of plan
    case histories, 91-92
    PowerPoint, 85-87
    secrets of successful, 87-91
    writing for success, 83-85
  survivor syndrome, 124-126
Dumbsizing, 11

"Effect of Online Literature Searching on Length of Stay and Patient Care Costs" (Klein and Ross), 30-31
E-journals, 70
Electronic Gaming Monthly (EGM), 65
Employee Assistance Program (EAP), 56
Employee Retirement Income Security Act (ERISA), 112
E-print archives, 70-71
E-reserve program, 71
Evaluation surveys, 29-30

Feedback form, 102
Fiscal studies, 27-29
Flowcharts, 29-30
"For Expert Literature Searching, Call a Librarian" (McGowan), 30
Full text, 69
Future Shock (Toffler), 5

Giuliani, Rudy, 65
The Godfather, Part I (motion picture), 39
Ground Rules for Winners: 12 Keys to Managing Team Players, Tough Bosses, Setbacks, and Success (Torre), 65
Gutenberg, Johannes, 5

Hammond, Patricia, 33
Health care, effect of changes in, 6-9
Homan, J. M., 31
Hospital libraries, unique problems of, 8
"Hospital Libraries Are an Economically Sound Investment" (Hammond and Priddy), 33

"The Hospital Library Is Crucial to Quality Healthcare" (Palmer), 32
Hospitals, as corporations, 4

"If" (Kipling), 133-134
"The Impact of the Hospital Library on Clinical Decision Making: The Rochester Study" (Marshall), 31
Implementation, of plan
 backpedaling, 100-101
 change, 93-95
 conflict resolution, 102-104
 layoffs, 98-99
 mergers, 96-97
 outsourcing, 95-96
 retraining staff, 97-98
 uh-oh factor, 100-101
In Search of Excellence (Peters), 2
Inner circle, and positioning, 62-66
Intelligence-gathering, 35-36
Internet, 3, 35
Interviews, 117-120

Joint Commission on Accreditation of Healthcare Organizations (JCAHO), 8, 26
Just-in-time hiring, 124

Ketchup packet affair, 14-15
Khrushchev, Nikita, 19
The Killer Angels (Shaara), 64, 65
King, D. N., 31-32
Kipling, Rudyard, 133-134
Kissinger, Henry, 17
Klein, M. S., 30-31
Kuhn, Thomas, 5

Lamb, Gertrude, 33
Layoffs, 98-99

Leadership, 20-21
Leadership (Giuliani), 65
Li, Jet, 53
Library staff
    communicating with, 47-49
    as tribe, 49-53
Liddy, G. Gordon, 91
Lightfoot, Gordon, 105
Lindberg, D. A., 32
Literature, 30-34
Louis XVI, 67

Machiavelli, 45
Malpractice, 7-8
Managed care companies, 8
Management style, 24
Marshall, J. G., 31
McGowan, J., 30
Medical technology, 7
Medicare, 6-7
MEDLINE, 30-31
Mergers, 12, 96-97
"Minimum Standards for Health
        Sciences Libraries" (Medical
        Library Association), 25, 26
Mission statement, 21-24
"Mn/DOT Library Accomplishments"
        (Baldwin), 33

Nietzsche, Frederick, 121

Online Computer Library Center
        (OCLC), 69-70
Organizational charts, 29-30
Outsourcing, 95-96

Palmer, R. A., 32
Paradigm shift
    defined, 5
    in medical libraries, 1-4, 5-6
    recognizing, 5-6
    in Swiss watch industry, 6

PC Magazine, 65
Personal digital assistants (PDAs), 68,
        69-70
Peters, Tom, 2
Phony War syndrome (PWS)
    business model, 61-62
    case histories, 58-60
    explained, 55-58
    inner circle and positioning, 62-66
    opportunities from other librarians,
        60-61
    recognizing opportunities, 58
PowerPoint, 85-87
Presentation, of plan
    case histories, 91-92
    PowerPoint, 85-87
    secrets of successful, 87-91
        laser pointers, 89-90
        points to remember, 87-89, 90-91
        wireless mikes, 90
    writing for success, 83-85
Priddy, Margy, 33
The Prince (Machiavelli), 45
PWS. *See* Phony War syndrome (PWS)

Quality improvement (QI), 28

Rapp, B. A., 32
Reagan, Ronald, 91
Reengineering, 11-12
Regulations, 25-27
Rehabilitation services, 7
Reorganization, 11-12
Restructuring, 11-12
Résumé, 18-20
Rightsizing, 11, 123
"The Role of Medical Librarians in
        Reducing Medical Errors"
        (Homan), 31
Ross, F. V., 30-31

Schacher, L. F., 32
Schott, Michael J., 1, 2, 17, 121

Seinfeld, Jerry, 55
Severance package, 12, 109-112
Shaara, Michael, 64, 65
Shakespeare, William, 83, 91, 93
Siegal, E. R., 32
Smith, Oliver, 58
Snoopy's Guide to the Writing Life
    (Conrad and Schulz), 65
Stealth downsizing, 11
Stengel, Casey, 67
Stewart, Martha, 65
The Structure of Scientific Revolution
    (Kuhn), 5
Survivor syndrome, 124-126
Swiss watch industry, 6
SWOT (strengths, weaknesses,
    opportunities, threats)
    analysis, 23
  opportunities, 74-75
  strengths, 73
  threats, 75
  weaknesses, 73-74

Toffler, Alvin, 5
Torre, Joe, 65
Truman, Harry, 105
Tzu, Sun, 3, 55, 120

Uh-oh factor, 100-101
Universal health care system, 8
"Use of MEDLINE by Physicians for
    Clinical Problem Solving"
    (Lindberg et al.), 32

Vision statement, 71-72

Wallingford, K. T., 32
Way of the weasel, 18
Wilson, S. R., 32
Worker Adjustment and Retraining
    Notification Act (WARN),
    112

Haworth Medical Information Sources
Sandra Wood, MLS, MBA
Senior Editor

BIOMEDICAL ORGANIZATIONS: A WORLDWIDE GUIDE TO POSITION DOCUMENTS by Dale A. Stirling. (2005).

MEDICAL LIBRARY DOWNSIZING: ADMINISTRATIVE, PROFESSIONAL, AND PERSONAL STRATEGIES FOR COPING WITH CHANGE by Michael J. Schott. (2005). "Michael Schott is fresh, funny, and fearless in this take-no-prisoners guide to dealing with corporate takeovers, mergers, and downsizing that threaten and challenge the survival of hospital libraries." *Elizabeth Connor, MLS, AHIP, Assistant Professor of Library Science, The Citadel, Charleston, South Carolina*

THE HERBAL INTERNET COMPANION: HERBS AND HERBAL MEDICINE ONLINE by David J. Owen. (2002). "Finally, someone has written a concise, referenced, unbiased, and thorough guide to navigating the Internet for information on herbs. This book is knowledgeable and factual, avoiding hyperbole, and plunging straight for the truth. . . . I consider this book an absolute must for anyone, professional or lay, seeking meaningful sources of herbal information on the Internet." *Paul L. Schiff Jr., PhD, Professor of Pharmaceutical Sciences, University of Pittsburgh*

HEALTH CARE RESOURCES ON THE INTERNET: A GUIDE FOR LIBRARIANS AND HEALTH CARE CONSUMERS edited by M. Sandra Wood. (2000). "A practical guide and an essential research tool to the Internet's vast and varied resources for health care has arrived—and its voice is professional and accessible . . . This comprehensive work is an important reference tool that is readable and enjoyable." *Elizabeth (Betty) R. Warner, MSLS, AHIP, Coordinator of Information Literacy Programs, Academic Information Services and Research, Thomas Jefferson University, Philadelphia, Pennsylvania*

EATING POSITIVE: A NUTRITION GUIDE AND RECIPE BOOK FOR PEOPLE WITH HIV/AIDS by Jeffrey T. Huber and Kris Riddlesperger. (1998). "Four stars! . . . A much-needed book that could have a positive impact on the quality of life for persons with HIV/AIDS. . . . Many of the recipes are old favorites that have been enhanced for the person with HIV. . . . All people with nutritional problems may also find this book helpful. It is not reserved solely for the person with HIV/AIDS." *Doody Publishing, Inc.*

HIV/AIDS AND HIV/AIDS-RELATED TERMINOLOGY: A MEANS OF ORGANIZING THE BODY OF KNOWLEDGE by Jeffrey T. Huber and Mary L. Gillaspy. (1996). "Provides the needed standardized terminology to describe large HIV/AIDS collections. . . . A welcome book for any cataloger, indexer, or archivist who is faced with organizing a mass of information that is growing very rapidly. . . . highly recommended for all librarians with extensive collections." *Booklist: Reference Books Bulletin*

HIV/AIDS COMMUNITY INFORMATION SERVICES: EXPERIENCES IN SERVING BOTH AT-RISK AND HIV-INFECTED POPULATIONS by Jeffrey T. Huber. (1996). "Provides a well-organized introduction to HIV/AIDS information services that will be useful to those affected by HIV disease, health care practitioners, librarians, and other information professionals. Appropriate for all libraries and an excellent reference resource." *CHOICE*

USER EDUCATION IN HEALTH SCIENCES LIBRARIES: A READER edited by M. Sandra Wood. (1995). "A welcome addition to any health sciences library collection. A valuable tool for both academic and hospital librarians, as well as library school students interested in bibliographic instruction." *National Network*

CD-ROM IMPLEMENTATION AND NETWORKING IN HEALTH SCIENCES LIBRARIES edited by M. Sandra Wood. (1993). "Neatly compacts information about the history, selection, and management of CD-ROM technology in libraries. . . . Librarians at all levels of CD-ROM implementation can benefit from the solutions and ideas presented." *Bulletin of the Medical Library Association*

HOW TO FIND INFORMATION ABOUT AIDS, SECOND EDITION edited by Jeffrey T. Huber. (1992). "Since organizations and sources in this field are constantly changing, this updated edition is welcome. . . . A valuable resource for health or medical and public library collections." *Booklist: Reference Books Bulletin*

Order a copy of this book with this form or online at:
http://www.haworthpress.com/store/product.asp?sku=5299

MEDICAL LIBRARY DOWNSIZING
Administrative, Professional, and Personal Strategies for Coping with Change

_____ in hardbound at $29.95 (ISBN: 0-7890-0413-5)

_____ in softbound at $19.95 (ISBN: 0-7890-0420-8)

Or order online and use special offer code HEC25 in the shopping cart.

COST OF BOOKS_____

☐ **BILL ME LATER:** (Bill-me option is good on US/Canada/Mexico orders only; not good to jobbers, wholesalers, or subscription agencies.)

☐ Check here if billing address is different from shipping address and attach purchase order and billing address information.

POSTAGE & HANDLING_____
(US: $4.00 for first book & $1.50 for each additional book)
(Outside US: $5.00 for first book & $2.00 for each additional book)

Signature_____

SUBTOTAL_____

☐ **PAYMENT ENCLOSED: $_____**

IN CANADA: ADD 7% GST_____

☐ **PLEASE CHARGE TO MY CREDIT CARD.**

STATE TAX_____
(NJ, NY, OH, MN, CA, IL, IN, & SD residents, add appropriate local sales tax)

☐ Visa ☐ MasterCard ☐ AmEx ☐ Discover
☐ Diner's Club ☐ Eurocard ☐ JCB

Account # _____

FINAL TOTAL_____
(If paying in Canadian funds, convert using the current exchange rate, UNESCO coupons welcome)

Exp. Date_____

Signature_____

Prices in US dollars and subject to change without notice.

NAME_____

INSTITUTION_____

ADDRESS_____

CITY_____

STATE/ZIP_____

COUNTRY_____ COUNTY (NY residents only)_____

TEL_____ FAX_____

E-MAIL_____

May we use your e-mail address for confirmations and other types of information? ☐ Yes ☐ No
We appreciate receiving your e-mail address and fax number. Haworth would like to e-mail or fax special discount offers to you, as a preferred customer. **We will never share, rent, or exchange your e-mail address or fax number.** We regard such actions as an invasion of your privacy.

Order From Your Local Bookstore or Directly From
The Haworth Press, Inc.
10 Alice Street, Binghamton, New York 13904-1580 • USA
TELEPHONE: 1-800-HAWORTH (1-800-429-6784) / Outside US/Canada: (607) 722-5857
FAX: 1-800-895-0582 / Outside US/Canada: (607) 771-0012
E-mailto: orders@haworthpress.com

For orders outside US and Canada, you may wish to order through your local sales representative, distributor, or bookseller.
For information, see http://haworthpress.com/distributors

(Discounts are available for individual orders in US and Canada only, not booksellers/distributors.)

PLEASE PHOTOCOPY THIS FORM FOR YOUR PERSONAL USE.
http://www.HaworthPress.com

BOF04